Keto Diet After 50

Complete Step-by-Step Guide to Ketogenic Diet for Seniors, With Delicious Recipes and Meal Plans. Fix Your Metabolism, Lose Weight and Stay Healthy.

Loretta Jephson

© Copyright 2021 by Loretta Jephson. All right reserved.

The work contained herein has been produced with the intent to provide relevant knowledge and information on the topic on the topic described in the title for entertainment purposes only. While the author has gone to every extent to furnish up to date and true information, no claims can be made as to its accuracy or validity as the author has made no claims to be an expert on this topic. Notwithstanding, the reader is asked to do their own research and consult any subject matter experts they deem necessary to ensure the quality and accuracy of the material presented herein.

This statement is legally binding as deemed by the Committee of Publishers Association and the American Bar Association for the territory of the United States. Other jurisdictions may apply their own legal statutes. Any reproduction, transmission or copying of this material contained in this work without the express written consent of the copyright holder shall be deemed as a copyright violation as per the current legislation in force on the date of publishing and subsequent time thereafter. All additional works derived from this material may be claimed by the holder of this copyright.

The data, depictions, events, descriptions and all other information forthwith are considered to be true, fair and accurate unless the work is expressly described as a work of fiction. Regardless of the nature of this work, the Publisher is exempt from any responsibility of actions taken by the reader in conjunction with this work. The Publisher acknowledges that the reader acts of their own accord and releases the author and Publisher of any responsibility for the observance of tips, advice, counsel, strategies and techniques that may be offered in this volume.

Table of Contents

Introduction 7

Chapter 1: Keto Diet Basics 9

    What Keto Means to You 9

    Keto & Your Daily Carbs 9

    Ketogenic Technique Levels 10

    What to Limit or Avoid 10

Chapter 2: Keto Diet At 50 & Beyond 17

    What Happens To Your Body? 17

    Supplements For Keto After 50 20

Chapter 3: The Keto Flu & Side Effects 22

Chapter 4: Keto Diet Benefits 26

Chapter 5: Keto Breakfast Recipes 28

    Smoothies & Beverages 28

        Bulletproof Hot Chocolate 28

        Healthy Green Smoothie 30

        Tasty Turmeric Milkshake 31

        Thai Iced Tea 32

        Vegan Bulletproof Coffee 33

        Coffee Creamer - Mint Chocolate 34

    Breakfast Goodies 35

        Apple Pie Pancakes 35

        Avocado Smoothie with Matcha 37

        Avocado Protein Smoothie 38

        Cinnamon Roll Muffins 39

        Crumbly Blueberry Bars 40

        Crust-Free Mini Quiche 42

        Low-Carb Maple "Oatmeal" 44

        Overnight Vanilla "Oatmeal" 45

        Tasty Tofu Scramble 46

Chapter 6: Lunch Favorites 47

Salad Option 47
- *Arugula Salad with Cherry Tomatoes* 47
- *Grab & Go Jar Salad* 49
- *Greek Chopped Salad* 50
- *Kale Salad* 51

Soup 52
- *Avocado Mint Chilled Soup* 52
- *Carrot Onion & Beef Soup - Instant Pot* 53
- *Chicken "Zoodle" Soup* 55
- *Superfood Soup* 56
- *Warm Vegan Walnut Chili* 57

Pasta Options 59
- *Asian BBQ Meatball Noodles Bowl* 59
- *Baked Zucchini Noodles With Feta* 61
- *Delicious Marinara Zoodles* 62
- *Fettuccine Chicken Alfredo* 63
- *Healthy Edamame Kelp Noodles* 65
- *Peanut Red Curry Vegan Bowl - Thai-Inspired* 66
- *Zucchini Lasagna* 67
- *Zucchini Noodle Alfredo - Vegan-Friendly* 68

Chapter 7: Keto Dinners 69

Poultry 69
- *Bruschetta Chicken* 69
- *Creamy Instant Pot Chicken* 70
- *French Garlic Chicken* 71
- *Lemon Rotisserie Chicken* 72
- *Whole Chicken & Gravy* 74

Pork 75
- *Carnitas* 75
- *Chipotle Pork Roast* 76

Pork Ribs *77*

Spicy Pork – Korean Style *80*

Beef 81

Bacon Burger Cabbage Stir Fry *81*

Beef Stroganoff *82*

Greek Meatballs with Tomato Sauce *84*

Italian Meatballs *85*

Shepherd's Pie *87*

Steak & Cheese Pot Roast *88*

Other Favorites 89

Mutton Curry *89*

Chapter 8: Keto Sides & Snacks 90

Sides 90

Baked Zucchini Noodles With Feta *90*

Cauliflower Fried "Rice" *91*

Crispy Cauliflower Zucchini Fritters *93*

Pad Thai with Zucchini Noodles *94*

Roasted Cabbage With Lemon *95*

Spaghetti Squash with Tomato & Mushroom *96*

Tofu Fries - Keto-Friendly *98*

Snacks 99

Baked Zucchini Chips *99*

Cauliflower Hummus with Garlic *101*

Delicious Guacamole *102*

Keto Seed Crackers *103*

Lettuce Wraps with Hemp Seed & Ginger *105*

Low-Carb Almond Flour Crackers *106*

Slow-Cooker Granola *107*

Tasty Keto Vegan Granola *109*

Trail Mix with Coconut *110*

Chapter 9: Keto Desserts 111

Chocolate Avocado Ice Cream 111

Chocolate Avocado Pudding 112

Chocolate Fat Bombs 114

Crunchy Protein Bars 115

Energy Balls 116

Key Lime Bars 117

Lemon Fat Bombs 119

Magical Chocolate Chip Bars 120

Mint Chocolate Chip Vegan Ice Cream 121

Peanut Butter Truffles 122

Protein Shake - Chocolate 124

Vegan Chocolate Fudge 125

Chapter 10: Keto Basic 21-Day Meal Plan 126

Week One: 127

Week Two: 128

Week Three: 129

Conclusion 130

Introduction

Congratulations on purchasing *Keto Diet After 50*, and thank you for doing so. The following chapters will discuss the keto diet basics, life beyond 50 and keto, and the keto flu symptoms and the diet's benefits.

The keto lifestyle is a specific way of living that revolves around strict adherence to the ketogenic or keto diet. This diet plan has been in use for centuries in one way or another, dating back to the ancient Greeks' time. They were the first to report that the effects of certain diseases and conditions could be lessened, if not cured completely, by following a particular eating plan. One of the conditions they treated with dietary restrictions was epilepsy, known then as 'having fits.' They noted that people who suffered from 'fits' had much less of this if they followed a particular diet.

The twentieth century brought us the first modern study into the effects of diet on 'fits,' which had been named epilepsy by then. In a small study with a group of patients, doctors found they could restrict the number of seizures per day by having their patients follow a low-calorie, high-fat diet. Since this was before medication had been invented, the doctor's only recourse at the time was to work with a patient's diet and level of activity.

When further looking at the results of the study and trying to determine how it worked so well, scientists discovered that the high-fat diet caused people's bodies to produce three different chemical compounds that were water-soluble and were only found in the bodies of people who were sticking to a starvation diet or one that was high in fat and low in carbohydrates. The scientists called these chemical bodies 'ketone bodies,' thus, the term ketogenic or keto diet was created.

The earliest keto diets were widely varied in the ratio of proteins to fats consumed. The doctors got the idea to try the diet on epilepsy patients, again without using the calorie restrictions. This new plan allowed people to eat until they felt full as long as their meals consisted of many fats with a moderate amount of protein and a low amount of carbohydrates.

The recommendation then was that the carbohydrate intake would not exceed twenty grams per day of all the food a patient ate. This plan not only reduced the number of seizures, if not eliminating them, but it gave other beneficial side effects. Patients were able to sleep better for longer periods. They lost weight and felt better. Their alertness and attention spans were greatly increased, and children who followed the diet were much better behaved than before.

This diet was widely used as a treatment for epilepsy until the middle part of the twentieth century when medications for epilepsy were developed. Swallowing a spoon of liquid or a pill was much easier than following a diet that was so restrictive. It could be difficult to follow the diet if the foods were not readily available. Refrigeration was still not widely available during this time, and many people did not have access to fresh dairy products like milk and cheese. People who lived in the city might not have access to fresh eggs. Much of the population survived on a diet of veggies grown in the home garden and were the staple of the daily diet. As a medical treatment, the keto diet became less widely used until it was no longer taught in medical school and eventually became nothing more than a historical entry in medical history books.

In the nineteen sixties and nineteen seventies, people were very conscious of their appearance, with the newly expanding world of media that gave people access to fashion trends from all around the world. The bikini was the swimsuit all women wanted to wear. The new fad diets also made money as people followed them with guaranteed quick weight loss and a beautiful body.

The keto diet was rediscovered and once again enjoyed popularity. Several different versions were created by different people who touted themselves as experts and named these diets after themselves. But the keto diet came into favor during the nineteen nineties to help a little boy whose seizures were so severe that medicine did not alleviate them. His parents desperately searched for anything that would help their little boy, and they came across medical literature outlining the keto diet and how it was originally used to control epilepsy. The diet was the answer they needed for their son and his seizures. Almost immediately, he stopped having the life-threatening seizures that had plagued him since birth.

So they made a documentary telling their story, and the keto diet once again jumped into the forefront of popular methods for weight loss. People embraced the keto diet and were fascinated by how it could help them lose weight and improve their lives. Doctors' original studies had recorded notes that most people lost weight and maintained a healthy weight. So the newest weight-loss sensation was a diet that was originally developed to control seizures in children and adults.

The keto diet basics have been a way of life for our ancestors, who were hunter-gatherers. They gathered whatever fruits and vegetables they could find to supplement their diet's staple, which was the meat they hunted. Our ancestors' diet was heavily based on meat and fat, with an occasional berry or carrot thrown in.

Every generation since then has become more obese as our lifestyles become more sedentary, and our diets become more heavily oriented around carbohydrates. So what is it about the keto diet that makes it the perfect solution for weight loss and disease prevention? The cause of all of these marvelous side effects is a thing known as ketosis.

Chapter 1: Keto Diet Basics

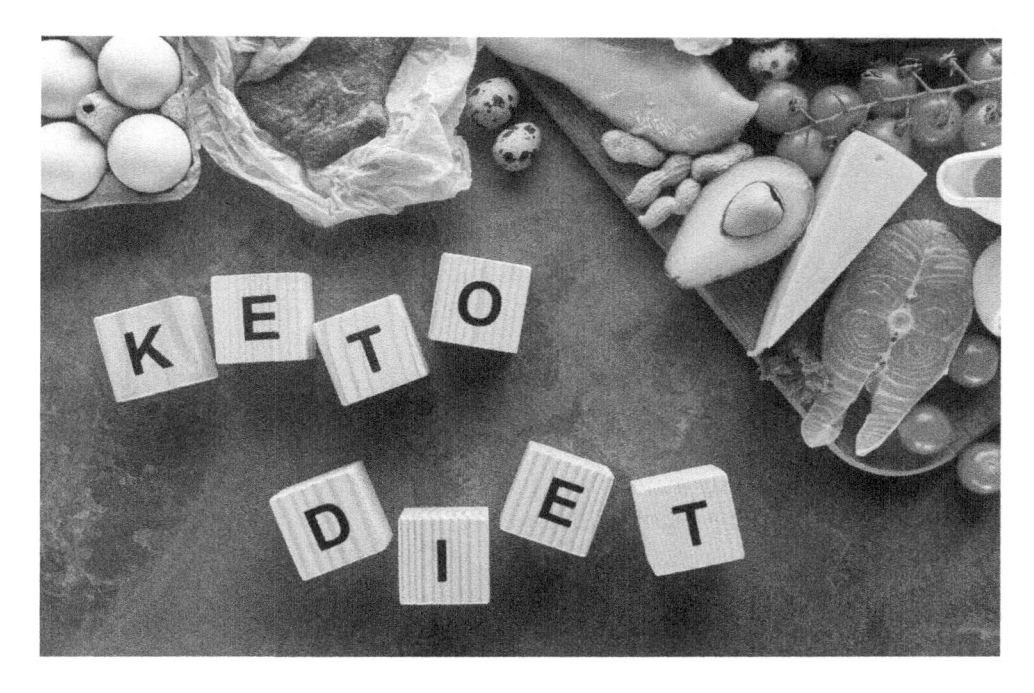

The ketogenic or keto diet is a low-carbohydrate, moderate protein, and higher fat diet plan that can help you burn fat more efficiently. Over fifty studies have shown its benefits for your health, weight loss, and performance, making it a recommended technique by an abundance of doctors. It can help you lose excess body fat without creating those nagging hunger bouts, as indicated in 2016 in the British Journal of Nutrition.

What Keto Means to You

Your body produces ketones, which are small fuel molecules, which is an alternate fuel source for the body when your glucose (blood sugar) is in short supply.

If you are eating fewer calories and fewer carbs, your liver will produce ketones from the fat. The ketones are a fuel source throughout your body, notably for the brain. Your brain is a hungry organ that will consume tons of energy daily, and it can't operate on fat directly. It can only work with ketones or glucose. Ketosis is reached as your body enters a metabolic state when your body produces these ketones.

Before you begin your keto plan, there are several ways you can accomplish your goals, depending on your needs.

Keto & Your Daily Carbs

These are the basic guidelines to consider as you blaze the path on the ketogenic diet plan:

- *Ketogenic 0-20 Carbs Daily* is the lowest level of carbs related to a restrictive medical diet. The patient is restricted from 10 to 15 grams each day to ensure the proper ketosis levels remain.

- *Moderate 20-50 Daily Carbs Allowed* if you have diabetes, are obese or are metabolically deranged, this is the plan for you. If you consume less than 50 grams daily, your body will achieve a ketosis state that supplies the ketone bodies.

- *Liberal 50-100 Daily Carbs Allowed* is the best incentive if you're active and lean and attempting to maintain your weight.

As you now see, it is vital to experiment and categorize where you fall on the scales before you make any changes. As with any new diet changes, you should seek your doctor's advice. You will soon realize the keto diet is flexible - yet strict. Each individual will lose weight differently, and other people may not have the same goals as you. For now, as a beginner, you will be using the first method.

Ketogenic Technique Levels

The standard ketogenic diet (SKD) comprises moderate protein, high fat, and low in carbs. The averages vary, but the ratio usually operates using 5% on carbs, 75% for high-fat, and 20% for your protein counts.

The targeted keto diet, which is also called TKD, will provide you with a technique to add carbs to the diet plan while working out or are more active.

The cyclical ketogenic diet (CKD) entails a restricted five-day keto diet plan followed by two high-carbohydrate days and is mostly adopted by athletes. This diet plan allows you to have meals rich in fats during most days of the week with just one or two cheat days where you eat meals with high-carb content. You need to adhere to this routine to achieve the most out of a keto diet.

The high-protein keto diet is comparable to the standard keto plan (SKD) in all aspects, except you will consume more protein.

Research has indicated that "unlike other low-carb diets, which focus on protein, a keto plan centers on fat, which supplies as much as 90% of your daily calories." Since there's no set rule for carb intake, you will want to be sure you are consuming the right amounts of food to keep your diet balanced for ketosis. You will be gradually working your way through the plan by eating plenty of vegetables, minimal intake of carbs, and two to three fruit pieces daily.

What to Limit or Avoid

The key to the ketogenic diet is balance. The foods listed in this segment are foods you should avoid or use as directed in ketogenic recipes.

Processed Foods:

Don't purchase any items if you see carrageenan on the label. Generally, look for labels with the least amount of ingredients. Usually, the ones that provide the most nutrition are listed in those shorter lists. These are just a few examples of processed snacks to avoid while on a ketogenic diet.:

- Crackers
- Rice Cakes
- Cereal Bars
- Popcorn
- Flavored Nuts
- PretzelsPotato Chips
- Protein Bars

The keto diet is restrictive, so unless you follow a prepared recipe, you will want to limit some of the following groups once you start to calculate your meal plans.

Sugars:

- Raw Sugar: 12 grams of carbs - 0 protein - 0 grams fat
- Agave Nectar: 14 grams of carbs - 0 protein or fat
- Honey: 17 grams of carbs - 0 protein or fat
- Maple Syrup: 14 grams of carbs - 0 protein or fat
- Cane Sugar: 12 grams of carbs - 0 protein or fat
- High-fructose Corn Syrup: 14 grams of carbs - 0 protein or fat
- Turbinado Sugar: 12 carbs - 0 protein or fat

Grains:

First, you need to realize grains are made from carbohydrates. This list is based on one cup servings. Avoid bread, pasta, pizza crusts, or crackers and cookies made with these grains unless indicated in a ketogenic recipe:

- Buckwheat: 33 carbs - 6 protein - 1 gram fat
- Wheat: (1 slice wheat bread) 14 carbs - 3 protein - 1 gram fat
- Barley: 44 carbs - 4 protein - 1 gram fat
- Quinoa: 39 carbs - 8 protein - 4 grams fat
- Corn: 32 carbs - 4 protein - 1 grams fat
- Millet: 41 carbs - 6 protein - 2 grams fat
- Bulgur: 33 carbs - 5.6 protein - 0.4 grams fat
- Amaranth: 46 carbs - 9 protein - 4 grams fat
- Oats: 36 carbs - 6 protein - 3 grams fat
- Rice: 45 carbs - 5 protein - 2 grams fat
- Rye: 15 carbs - 3 protein - 1 gram fat

Beans & Legumes:

- Kidney Beans: 18.5 carbs - 7 protein - 0.75 grams fat
- Black Beans: 23 carbs -7 protein - 0.5 grams fat
- Chickpeas: 20 carbs - 6 protein - 2 grams fat
- Lentils: 19 carbs - 8 protein - 0 grams fat
- White Beans/Great Northern: 22 carbs - 8 protein - 0 grams fat
- Green Peas: 14 carbs - 4 protein - 0 grams fat
- Lima Beans: carbs - protein - grams fat
- Cannellini Beans: carbs - protein - grams fat
- Black Eyed Peas: 14 carbs - 2 protein - 0 grams fat
- Fava Beans: 17 carbs - 2 protein - 0 grams fat

Starchy Vegetables:

- Yams: 19 carbs - 1 protein -0 grams fat
- Sweet Potatoes: 14 carbs - 1 protein - 0 grams fat
- Potatoes (1 medium baked) 28 carbs - 3 protein - 0.3 grams fat
- Carrots: 6 carbs - 1 protein - 0 grams fat
- Corn: 32 carbs - 4 protein - 1 gram fat
- Peas: 14 carbs - 4 protein - 0 grams fat
- Yucca (.5 cup raw) 39 carbs - 1.5 protein - 0 grams fat

Fruits:

- Apples – no skin - boiled – 13.6 total carbs
- Apricots - 7.5 total carbs
- Bananas - 23.4 total carbs
- Fresh Blackberries - 5.4 net carbs
- Fresh Blueberries - 8.2 net carbs
- Fresh Strawberries - 3 net carbs
- Cantaloupe - 6 total carbs
- Raw Cranberries - 4 net carbs
- Gooseberries - 8.8 net carbs
- Kiwi – 14.2 total carbs
- Fresh Boysenberries - 8.8 net carbs
- Oranges – 11.7 total carbs
- Peaches - 11.6 total carbs
- Pears – 19.2 total carbs
- Pineapple - 11 total carbs
- Plums – 16.3 total carbs
- Watermelon -7.1 total carbs

Keep in mind; these are merely estimates so you recognize how easily carbs can hide in typically 'healthy' foods. Let's take this one step further. It is essential to maintain your health using fresh, raw, or organic milk products. It is also vital to purchase full-fat dairy items. The harder cheeses usually have fewer carbs. You can also add additional protein and calcium using non-dairy products, including almond, coconut, or cashew milk.

These are a few of the products used to stock your fridge and their nutritional values:

- Soft and hard cheeses (ex. sharp cheddar or mozzarella)
- Brie Cheese - 0.1 grams - net carbs per 1 oz.
- Colby/Cheddar cheese - 0.4 net carbs per 1 oz.
- Cottage cheese - 2% fat - 4.1 per .5 cup
- Cottage cheese - creamed - 2.8 per .5 cup
- Heavy whipping cream - double cream - whipped - 3 grams of net carbs per .5 cup
- Cream cheese - 0.8 net carbs per 2 tbsp.
- Sour cream - 1 gram net carb per 1 tbsp.
- Feta Cheese - 1.2 grams net carbs per 1 oz.
- Parmesan cheese - 0.9 per 1 oz.

Keto-Friendly Sweeteners

Stevia Drops offer delicious flavors, including hazelnut, vanilla, English toffee, and chocolate. Some individuals think the drops are too bitter, so at first, use three drops to equal one teaspoon of sugar.

Xylitol is at the top of the sugary list as an excellent choice to sweeten your teriyaki and barbecue sauce and teriyaki. Its natural-occurring sugar alcohol has a Glycemic index (GI) standing of 13.

Swerve Granular Sweetener is also an excellent choice as a blend. It's made from non-digestible carbs sourced from starchy root veggies and select fruits. Start with 3/4 of a teaspoon for every one of sugar. Increase the portion to your taste.

The best all-around sweetener is Pyure Organic All-Purpose Blend. There's no bitter aftertaste with this stevia-based product. The blend of stevia and erythritol is an excellent alternative to your sweetening, baking, and cooking needs. It is suggested that you substitute 1/3 teaspoon of Pyure for every one teaspoon of sugar. Adjust this to your taste since you can always add a bit more.

For powdered sugar, you can grind the sweetener in a NutriBullet or other blender until it's very dry.

Sukrin Gold provides a brown sugar alternative. The mixture of stevia and erythritol claims the one-to-one ratio for sugar. It is always best to start with the rate of ¾ of a teaspoon per one teaspoon of sugar. According to the United States standards, this is not a good choice if you are seeking a gluten-free alternative because it contains malt extract.

Lakanto provides an apple-flavored - sugar-free syrup with a monk-fruit and erythritol based. You can also select the *Golden Monk Fruit Sweetener* as a brown sugar choice. The name monk-fruit came from the Buddhist monks over 1,000 years ago. It is considered a cooling-agent and may not agree with your digestive system. Use it sparingly if using baked goods.

Excellent Spices

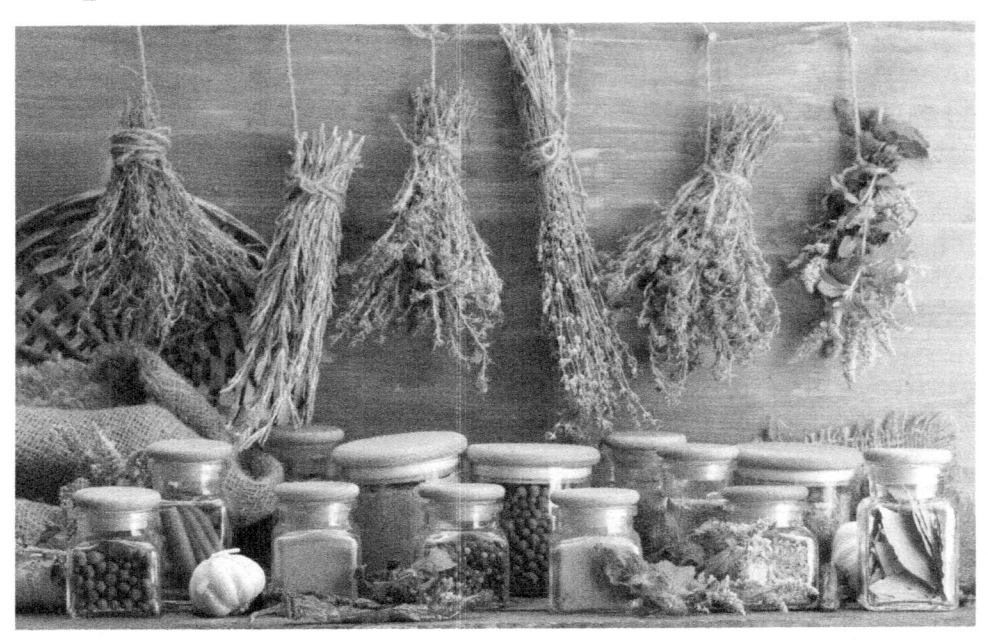

Planning ahead of time on your ketogenic diet means you will be counting the carbs in the food you're planning to prepare. If you're starting from scratch and not using a recipe, you will want to know how many carbs you consume for each portion. These are a few of the popular spices used so you'll have an idea the next time you go to shake or chop:

- Salt – .0 grams
- Basil - .3 grams
- Cinnamon – .6 grams
- Garlic Powder – 1.0 gram
- Nutmeg – .6 grams
- Oregano – .1 grams
- Paprika – .4 grams
- Rosemary – .2 grams
- Thyme – .3 grams
- Dill – .4 grams

Black Pepper: Pepper promotes nutrient absorption in the tissues all over your body, speeds up your metabolism, and improves digestion. The main ingredient of pepper is a pipeline, which gives it a pungent taste. It can boost fat metabolism by as much as 8% for up to several hours after it's ingested. As you will see, it is used throughout your ketogenic recipes, hailing at zero grams.

Cinnamon: Use cinnamon as part of your daily plan to improve your insulin receptor activity. Just put one-half of a teaspoon of cinnamon into a smoothie, shake, or a keto dessert. As you observe, many of the keto recipes contain the ingredient.

Cayenne Pepper: The secret ingredient in cayenne is capsaicin, a natural compound that gives the peppers their fiery heat. This provides a slight increase in your metabolism. The peppers are also rich in vitamins, useful as an appetite controller, smooths out digestion issues, and benefit your heart health.

Turmeric: The use of this Asian orange herb dates back to Ayurveda and Chinese medicine. Curcumin is an anti-inflammatory compound found in turmeric. It helps improve your insulin receptor function while regulating your blood sugar levels. It aids in digestion and improves weight management. Add turmeric to your meats, vegetables, green drinks, or smoothies. To maximize the antioxidant elements, add the turmeric after the meal has finished cooking.

Mustard Seed: Spicy mustard can help boost your metabolism and allow you to burn fat quickly because of its thermogenic properties. Try substituting mayonnaise with mustard. They have the same creamy texture, and you'll only be spending about one-tenth of the calories.

Choose Healthy Oils & Fats

Coconut Oil: You vamp up the fat intake with this high flash-point oil. Enjoy a coconut oil smoothie before your workouts. Use it with your meats, chicken, fish, or on top of veggies. It will quickly transfer from solid form to oil according to its temperature.

Extra-Virgin Olive Oil (EVOO): Olive oil dates back for centuries – back to when priests and kings were anointed using pure oil. High-quality oil with its low-acidity makes the oil have a smoke point as high as 410° Fahrenheit. That's higher than most cooking applications call for, making olive oil more heat-stable than many other cooking fats. It contains (2 tsp.) -0- carbs.

Monounsaturated fats, such as the ones in olive oil, are also linked with better blood sugar regulation, including lower fasting glucose and reducing inflammation throughout the body. Olive oil also helps prevent cardiovascular disease by protecting your vascular system's integrity and lowering LDL, also called the 'bad cholesterol.

Keto-Friendly Monounsaturated & Saturated Fats:

Include these items (listed in grams):

- Olives 10 small – 3 jumbo - 5 large – 1 net carb
- Chicken fat/Duck Fat/Beef Tallow – 1 tbsp. - 0 net carbs
- Unsweetened flaked coconut – 3 tbsp. – 2 net carbs
- Unsalted Butter/Ghee – 1 tbsp. -0 net carbs
- Egg yolks – 1 large – 0.6 net carbs
- Organic Red Palm oil – ex. Nutiva - 1 tbsp. -0- net carbs
- Avocado oil/Sesame oil – 1 tbsp. - 0 net carbs
- Flaxseed oil – 1 tbsp. – 0 net carbs
- Various Dressings
- Keto-Friendly Mayonnaise

Chapter 2: Keto Diet At 50 & Beyond

The ketogenic diet can provide many benefits, which you will discover in-depth in future chapters. First, let's explore how a woman's body reacts to aging. We will cover areas difficult for women and other individuals on the plan.

What Happens To Your Body?

Many women are entering menopause, but you need to understand the process as it has effects on all women:

- Restricting your carbs and calories too much on a keto diet can lead to out-of-balance hormones.

- Weight loss plateaus — or even weight gain — are a standard stumbling block for women on keto. One way to fight back is to incorporate more fat or try periods of intermittent fasting.

- Women who notice their energy is dragging should do carb cycling — "carb-up" once or twice a week with starchy vegetables.

- If emotional eating is thwarting your keto efforts, break habit loops by switching your routine in small ways.

- Ditching a deprivation mindset can help you reframe the narrative around your diet, enabling you to stick with it.

The Issues Explained Further

Your Short-Term Memory Changes: Have you ever been around an individual who is over 50? If you are close with that person, you may notice some of the short-term memories will begin to fade, which can impact your daily routines. It's often displayed in the form of slowed reaction times and poor judgment.

Your Brain May Weaken: Your brain is much like a muscle and must be used, or it will become weak and shrink. Do new things in your life and step out of your comfort zone. It pushes your brain into an active mode when you switch things up. It could be as simple as going down a different path on the way home or changing the way you eat! Break the routine and try intermittent fasting to help slow the aging process.

Your Metabolism Slows Down: The main element to remember is you need to take in fewer calories.

Your Skin Changes: You will experience a lack of estrogen, which affects your skin, making it have the appearance of cellulite more prevalent and crepe-like. You can use a remedy on the intermittent fasting plan. Have a bit of bone broth or a dash of collagen powder to a cup of coffee or smoothie.

Your Hair & Nails Become Stressed: It's vital to increase your calcium intake because, like your skin, your hair and nails also change. You may notice your nails are brittle, and your hair has a bunch of split ends.

You'll Have More Dental Issues: By the age of 50, your tooth enamel erodes, creating an increase in dental issues. The issues may require increased care to eliminate tooth pain and unwanted cavities. It's vital to have regular dental exams and stop some of the woes after 50!

Your Eyesight May Deteriorate or Weaken: As you age, the darkness may be your worst enemy, which increases the issues involved with depth and distance perception. It's probably not to drive except during daylight hours. It's essential to take care of your eyesight and visit your optician regularly.

You Are More Susceptible to Injuries: You don't think about injuries at 50 because your mindset still thinks it's as agile now as it was at 21. Unfortunately, you're more likely to suffer from medical issues like carpal tunnel syndrome, tendinitis, and plantar fasciitis. It's recommended to take frequent breaks if you're at a work desk all day. Exercise is the key, so stretch your forearms or develop another inventive way to keep your muscles active to avoid so many repetitive movements.

Hormonal Changes May Prompt Digestive Issues: As hormones change, expect the menopause changes (on average) by 51. It's possible you will suffer from gas, bloating, and constipation.

Your Muscle Loss Accelerates: Your peak of muscle mass generally occurs at the age of 25. After 50, the loss of hormones, such as the growth hormone, is reduced. Make adequate sleeping a goal since that's when your hormones are released. Opt for short intervals and weight training, working hard at short intervals, "hit it and quit it!"

Your Bone Loss Accelerates: The menopause time brings forth acceleration for three to five years, leading to bone fractures, many times brought on by a fall. Workout using your major muscle groups for some improvement of bone protection. Try working out a couple of times each week.

You Lose Flexibility: Don't try to do the splits as you did in your younger years. Your tendons and muscles lose their elasticity. Your spinal discs will also degenerate with age, raising your chances of injuries. You may need to use alternative healthcare as part of your health regimen. Consider chiropractic care, massage therapy, and stretching exercises.

Your Body Stores More Fat: Aging causes your body to store fat readily and reluctantly burns fat, especially if you are dehydrated or stressed. Estrogen dropping adds to the adverse effects of stress. It also deviates the fat from reproductive areas. Thus, you gain weight around the belly - losing your hourglass figure. The intermittent fasting methods will assist you by providing snacks and treats to enjoy using the ketogenic dieting methods. Provide extra fiber and protein to reduce your cravings and keep you satiated longer.

Lactose Intolerance Becomes An Issue: Milk is considered the #1 calcium supplier for strong and healthy bones. Aging can bring forth problems with women digesting milk properly as she ages. Intermittent fasting can add back some of the calcium by providing your diet with leafy greens, Greek yogurt, hard cheese, kefir, and tofu.

Your Fat Will Redistribute: During child-bearing years, the woman's body has fat allocated to her thighs and hips to support carrying a child. That changes during menopause as the body produces less estrogen; the fat collects in the tummy area, called 'menopause belly.'

You May Develop Foot Conditions: Some individuals will have deformities, including bunions and hammertoes, as a part of the aging process. In some cases, they are hereditary. Choose a good-fitting shoe that's not too tight to dissuade the worsening of the problem.

Your Feet Will Change Shape: It sounds crazy, but you may notice your feet become wider or longer during the aging process. According to Dr. Petkov, a podiatrist in New Jersey, "They can grow half a size in a decade." Your feet can also become flat since the ligaments and tendons lose their resilience. You will find that weight is a huge factor. It's essential to have someone measure your feet every few years to ensure that you are buying the right shoe size.

Your Body Synthesizes Protein Less Effectively: After 50, it's essential to consume adequate protein in your diet, or muscle loss may result. Strength training can improve the process, so it's vital to enjoy a high-protein meal about one or two hours after you have your workout.

You Are More Prone To Calcium Deficiency: Your bones are weakened when calcium is depleted. The lack of calcium can lead to bone pain and tenderness or osteoporosis. You should ingest 1200 mg. of calcium daily. Once again, intermittent fasting using cheese and yogurt are excellent remedies. Other calcium-rich foods include kidney beans, kale, broccoli, oranges, sesame seeds, edamame, and almonds.

You Might Develop Dry Mouth: With aging, the possibilities of diabetes, high blood pressure, arthritis, and Parkinson's, many individuals suffer from dry mouth brought on by many of the popular medications used to treat the ailment. Dry mouth can also lead to fungal infections of the throat, tongue, and other areas, including tooth decay and gum disease. Drink lots of water to stay hydrated, ensuring you floss regularly to remove plaque and food possibly stuck in your teeth.

Your Libido Declines As You Go Through Menopause: Get plenty of sleep and opt for strength training a couple of times each week. You should also perform short interval training sessions once or twice weekly. Reducing the amount of sugar and alcohol (if you drink) you consume can boost your libido.

Supplements For Keto After 50

It is advisable to consult your regular physician before you begin the diet plan. The doctor can advise you concerning which nutrients may need replacement if you do not like the types of foods you should eat.

Many individuals will experience headaches, fatigue, or nausea - sometimes called 'induction flu.' As you remove the carbs, your potassium and sodium (vital electrolytes) are also removed. Taking a supplement will help with these issues, even if you are not over 50.

Greens/Veggie Supplements: You need to get the greens in your keto diet by enjoying spinach, have a salad with dinner, or other meals with greens. However, if you don't like greens, you can purchase a greens supplement. A measuring scoop of a protein shake will help with the issue.

CoQ10 or Coenzyme Q10: Coenzyme Q10 is the technical term for this powerful antioxidant. It is also a central molecule in your cellular process of creating energy. You can supplement your diet with 100 to 300 mg each day.

Glutamine: Eight grams daily—taken orally—immediately after your workout—can help promote glucose production during exercise. When you purchase glutamine, don't buy the powders because they usually have additives or sugar content.

Probiotics: You can eat kimchi (sometimes spelled kimchi), Greek yogurt, kefir, or similar fermented foods, or you can take a supplement.

Electrolytes: You may experience headaches, fatigue, or nausea, sometimes called 'induction flu.' As you remove the carbs, your potassium and sodium (essential electrolytes) are also removed. Taking a supplement will help with these issues.

Malate or Magnesium Citrate Supplement: It is vital to assist your diet plan if you have constipation issues. Activate over 76% of the enzymatic processes in your body with a supplement. You can take between 400 to 600 mg each day.

Sodium Supplements: You should receive at least one to two grams of extra sodium daily. Some of the pros accomplish this with bouillon cubes. Sea Salt is a great option used in your diet plan. You should receive 3000 to 5000 mg of sodium daily.

Potassium Supplement: You can become low in potassium in the short-term because of the vomiting and diarrhea that could go along with your early stages to the keto plan. Natural potassium can also be received through milk, whole grains, bananas, veggies, peas, and beans. It's recommended for you to take supplements because potassium also leaves your body with salt. As part of your well-prepared meal plan, you should receive 3000 to 4000 mg of potassium daily.

Magnesium Supplement: For magnesium, 300-500 mg is an initial recommendation. Muscle cramps are your best indicator of depletion.

Vanadium and Chromium: Chromium and Vanadium are both trace minerals - essential to insulin production, which will stabilize your body's blood sugar level.

You can also use lemons and lime as a natural supplement. Lemon and Lime: Your blood sugar levels will naturally drop with these citric additions and signal a boost in your liver function. Use them in green juices, with a salad, or with cooked meat or veggies. The choices are limitless and assist you with the following:

- Excellent for weight loss
- Relieves respiratory infections
- Reduces toothache pain
- Boosts your immune system
- Balances pH
- Decreases wrinkles and blemishes
- Reduces fever
- Blood purifier
- Flushes out the unwanted, unhealthy materials

Chapter 3: The Keto Flu & Side Effects

Keto begins and ends with carb restriction. Restricting carbs sends your body into ketosis, which makes you shed excess body fat. And this is why the keto diet is so effective for so many people. You will experience a decrease in hunger and an increase in your energy levels. It will make it easier for you to consume fewer calories and lose weight naturally while improving your health.

You might experience some unpleasant side effects while you are getting used to the keto diet. You will need to be kind to yourself and give your body time to adapt to living the low-carb life. These side effects are quite worth it because soon, you will begin to enjoy each keto lifestyle benefit. Before you become discouraged and give up on your dreams of an ideal body and a healthy lifestyle, keep in mind that these symptoms, if you experience them, are temporary and will soon go away.

The ultimate goal of beginning and following the keto diet is entering a state of ketosis. This state will make your body burn stored fat for fuel instead of the food you consume. There are several factors involved in getting your body into ketosis. Among these factors is how restrictive your intake of carbs is. The difference between your weight when you start, and your desired weight is another factor. If you have severely restricted your caloric intake because you have considerable weight to lose, you might enter into ketosis quicker. If you have not greatly restricted your calories because you have a larger daily need, then you may need more time for your body to enter ketosis.

The keto diet will adjust how your metabolism works. The worst side effect of the keto diet is when you go through the keto flu. You can take the diet in small steps and ease into it rather than jump right into it. If you allow your body to adjust to the diet over a longer period of three to four weeks, you will go through ketosis more slowly. This method takes longer, but you will not have as many negative symptoms immediately after beginning.

Most people begin immediately and get ketosis over with - quickly to burn stored body fat. Using this method will give you results sooner rather than later, and immediate progress is often enough incentive to keep people following the diet when they feel like quitting.

When you enter ketosis, your body will radiate symptoms that will feel like you have the flu, often referred to as the keto flu. These symptoms will begin within two to five days after you start on the diet and last for one to two weeks. You might have some of these symptoms:

- Bad breath
- Bloating from water retention after a day of higher carb intake
- Constipation
- Headaches
- Increasing cravings, especially for sugary foods or carbs

- Loss of libido
- Moodiness or irritability
- Periods of low energy and exhaustion
- Sleeping disturbances
- Weakness during and after exercise

Ketosis can cause bad breath because waste products are being eliminated from your body. Your body will remove toxins through sweat, breathing, urination, and defecation. When toxins are coming out of your mouth, your breath will smell bad, and it will not matter how often you brush your teeth. Chewing a few sugar-free gum pieces will help with this symptom, and it will not last long.

When you begin following the keto diet, you might feel moody and irritable, and there is a simple explanation for that. When you eat carbohydrates, they almost immediately turn into sugar in your body during the process of digestion. It will not matter if the carb is a fruit, vegetable, or honey bun. Your body does not know the difference between bad food and good food. When you consume sugar, it just becomes sugar in your body. When your body detects an increase in your blood sugar level, your brain releases chemicals like dopamine and serotonin. These two chemicals make your brain feel increased happiness, and they provide a calming effect on your body. When you take the carbs out of your diet, the brain may stop producing these chemicals temporarily, and this can make you feel moody and irritable. These feelings will soon pass when your body adjusts to living on fewer carbs and more proteins and fats.

Decreased amounts of sugar in your bloodstream can also cause you to suffer from headaches. Imbalances can also cause these in the electrolytes in your body. It is especially important during the first few weeks of following keto to remain hydrated. You will need to help your body flush the toxins out. And maintaining a good balance of electrolytes is important, so you might want to add a bit of salt and sugar to your water or indulge in a few sugar-free sports drinks.

Your body will undergo many adjustments and changes as it learns to adjust to using fat for energy instead of using the glucose it normally uses. Your body will use all of the energy it has available to manage these processes. That may mean that you will have precious little extra energy for anything else. You may feel particularly exhausted if you are exercising during this time. It is good for you to exercise regularly, and it will help increase your weight loss; you might find you need to lighten up on your physical exertion for a short time during the time in which your body will be adjusting to your new food intake. You do not need to completely give up exercising; just switch to a less intense form of exercise that you like doing. Bicycling, swimming or walking are all excellent forms of exercise, and these will allow you to exercise at a slower pace, which you can easily handle during this time.

You might experience muscle weakness brought on by the change in your diet. You need to make sure that you are eating the recommended amount of protein on the keto diet. Your protein intake will be in the form of poultry, meat, eggs, or fish. You may also want to take a magnesium supplement to ensure your muscles stay strong. Adding a half teaspoon of some natural sea salt to eight ounces of water to help replenish the sodium you are losing through your waste products may also help. The production of waste will be increased as your body works to remove and discard the toxins out. A few teaspoons of lemon juice or lime juice will mask the taste of the salt.

When you begin the keto diet, you will naturally feel cravings for the foods you are no longer eating - this is a natural phase - because suddenly - you have cut a large group of items out of your diet that you have long been used to eating. You will be consuming enough of the right kind of food to curb your feelings of hunger. But this will not eliminate those cravings, especially for foods that are now off-limits to you. Cravings might just be an emotional response to knowing that you can't have a piece of pie or a donut. Find something to occupy your time when cravings hit to redirect your attention. They will go away in time.

You may suddenly develop problems sleeping well due to the sudden decrease in carbohydrates in your diet. The sudden lack of chemicals in the brain that brings you good feelings is why these are the same chemicals that make you sleepy, and the lack of them can cause an immediate disruption in sleep. Melatonin and serotonin are chemicals that are released by your brain when you consume carbs. Serotonin will make you happy, and melatonin will make you sleepy. Following the keto diet will eventually lead to better sleep patterns because it will regulate hormones' released into your body. While you are waiting for this to happen, try to take part in gentle exercise a few hours before going to bed, like gentle cycling or taking a long, slow walk around the neighborhood. These activities will help release those hormones that will make you feel happy and help relax your body and prepare you for a good night's sleep. Try to keep your sleep schedule the same, even on your days off work.

Constipation or bloating are both common occurrences at the beginning of the keto diet. You may also experience random bouts of diarrhea. You may be lucky enough to experience no gastrointestinal changes at all. Everyone's body is different, and food will affect everyone differently. Any constipation that you experience can be relieved if you stay hydrated well.

Warm water, or at the least room-temperature water, is the best choice for stimulating your digestive processes. It might help you if you add a few drops of lime or lemon juice to your water, as well as drinking hot water with lemon or lime in it. Herbal teas, black or green tea, black coffee, and broth will also help you either relieve constipation or ease the stomach upset that might come with diarrhea.

Keep reminding yourself that any negative effects of ketosis will last just a short time, but the positive effects of ketosis will last you as long as your body remains in the state of ketosis. And getting into ketosis is just the beginning of the good things that the keto diet will bring you. Following the keto diet will jump-start and promote weight loss. It is a lifestyle plan that you will maintain and incorporate into your daily life because it offers enough calories and fat to keep you feeling fuller longer. Your body will be forced to rely on your fat stores for fuel in the beginning since the keto diet is naturally low in carbs. And reducing your daily consumption of carbs will automatically result in an elimination of all of those empty calories that come from carbs. You will no longer be consuming those empty calories, so you will notice almost immediate weight loss as your body begins to consume its own stored fat.

Following the keto diet will suppress your hunger feelings and reduce any food cravings. As long as your body constantly stays in the state of ketosis, you will not need to measure your portions or count calories, especially if you do not go crazy and overeat. Most people who reach ketosis will find that their diet leaves them feeling satisfied longer on less food and more energized from their food choices.

Ketosis will regulate your appetite and lower your overall desire to eat. And the ketone bodies that are produced while your body is in ketosis will feed the region of the brain that houses the hypothalamus, which is the area that controls the rate of metabolism. Ketosis will not cause your metabolism to slow down, as most other diets do.

You will also feel an increased ability to focus and higher energy levels while you are in ketosis. Your body will become accustomed to burning ketones for fuel instead of relying on massive amounts of glucose. Your muscles will learn to prefer using ketones for energy. The protein that you eat will be used to feed those parts of the brain that require a bit of glucose to function properly.

The unpleasant side effects of adjusting to the keto diet will go away on their own as your body adjusts to all the changes in nutrition, and your hormones become unbalanced within the first few weeks. Keto flu symptoms can easily be managed by eating more fat, getting plenty of sleep, and staying well-hydrated with water and electrolytes. Be patient with yourself and your reactions because this will pass, and soon, you will begin to reap all the benefits the keto diet can offer you.

Chapter 4: Keto Diet Benefits

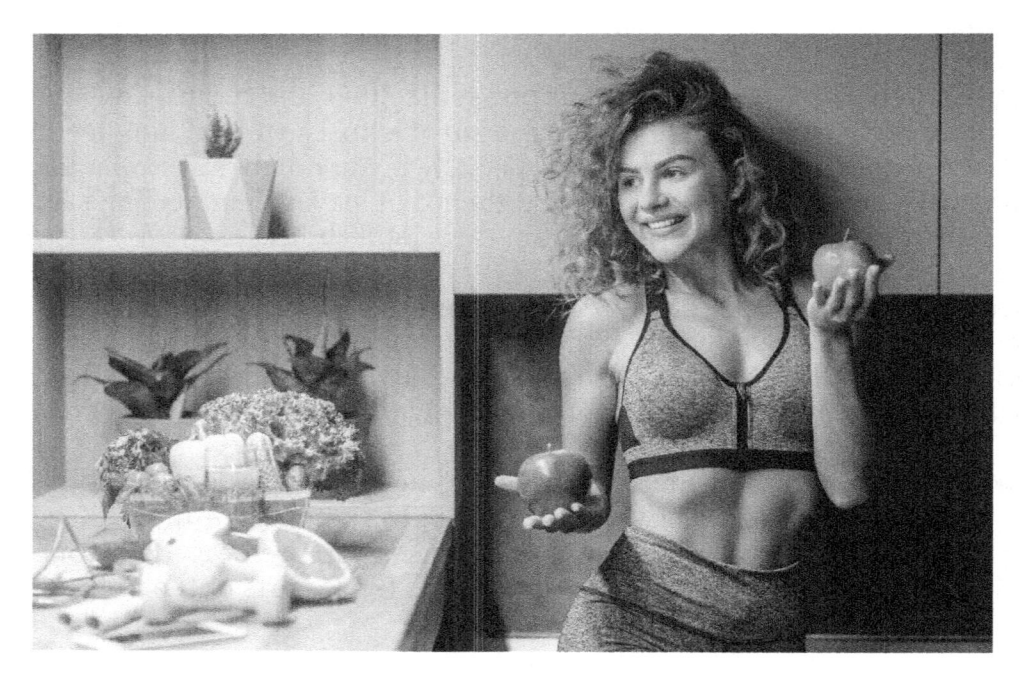

Even though the ketogenic diet plan is somewhat restrictive, it provides you with numerous benefits. These are some of the most prominent ones:

Accelerated Fat Loss for Overweight & Obese Individuals: Weight Loss And Anti-Aging is improved long term according to a Harvard Study in 2018. Those who participate in the keto's intermittent fasting phase diet plan may exceed healthy figures when it comes to weight. It is imperative to use the keto diet plan to get started on the right path for weight loss.

Improved Thinking Skills: Your brain is approximately 60% fat by weight. Therefore, you might become confused as you consume high-fat foods. By increasing your fatty food intake, you will have better chances to better your mind. It can maintain itself and work at full capacity.

Epileptic Seizures: For children, reductions in seizures have occurred for children who have used the keto diet. The therapeutic keto diet used for epilepsy often restricts the carbs to fewer than 15 grams of carbs daily to further escalate your ketone levels. Don't try to reach these levels unless you have the supervision of a medical professional.

Dravet Syndrome, a severe form of epilepsy, is marked by prolonged, uncontrollable, and frequent seizures. Currently, available medications don't improve symptoms in about 1/3 of the Dravet Syndrome patients. A clinical study used 13 children with the syndrome to stay on the ketogenic diet for more than one year to remain seizure-free. Over 50% of the group decreased in the frequency of the seizures. In conclusion, six of the patients stopped the diet later, and one remains seizure-free.

Improvement Of Your Cholesterol Profile: An arterial buildup is typically associated with triglyceride and cholesterol levels, proven to improve with the keto diet plan. Cut down your chance of heart disease. The triglycerides found in large amounts in carbohydrates are also found in high concentrations in those who have experienced cardiovascular problems.

Blood Pressure Levels Lowered: When you begin the ketogenic diet, your blood pressure may become lower, making you feel dizzy at first. Don't worry or feel overly concerned because that's a clear indication that the carbohydrates are working. However, suppose you are currently taking medications. It's a good idea to speak with your physician about the possibility of lowering some of your doses during the time that you are on the ketogenic plan.

Regulate Your Blood Sugar: According to a London 2005 Study, the ketogenic diet can help reduce the "bad" LDL cholesterol, inflammatory markers, blood triglycerides, and blood sugar for those with type 2 diabetes.

Polycystic Ovary Syndrome (PCOS) Improves: This is an endocrine disorder affecting young women of childbearing years. It is also associated with insulin resistance, obesity, and hyperinsulinemia. A 6-month study concluded a significant improvement in weight loss in fasting women over 24 weeks. The group limited carb intake to 20 grams daily for 24 weeks.

Alzheimer's Disease: The disease's progression can be slowed, and the symptoms reduced with the keto plan.

Cancer: Several types of cancer and slow tumor growths are being treated by using the keto diet technique.

Gum Disease and Tooth Decay: The pH balance in your mouth is influenced by sugar intake. Your gum issues could subside after about three months on a keto diet plan. You will be consuming healthier foods.

Acne: By eating fewer processed foods and less sugar, your insulin levels will be lowered, and acne outbreaks should improve.

Joint Pain and Stiffness: Grain-based foods are eliminated from your diet on the keto plan. It is believed the grains can be one of the biggest causes of pain or chronic illness. After all, it has been said before, "no pain –no grain."

Don't worry; the food is delicious when you use your step-by-step instructions for each recipe provided in your new cookbook.

Chapter 5: Keto Breakfast Recipes

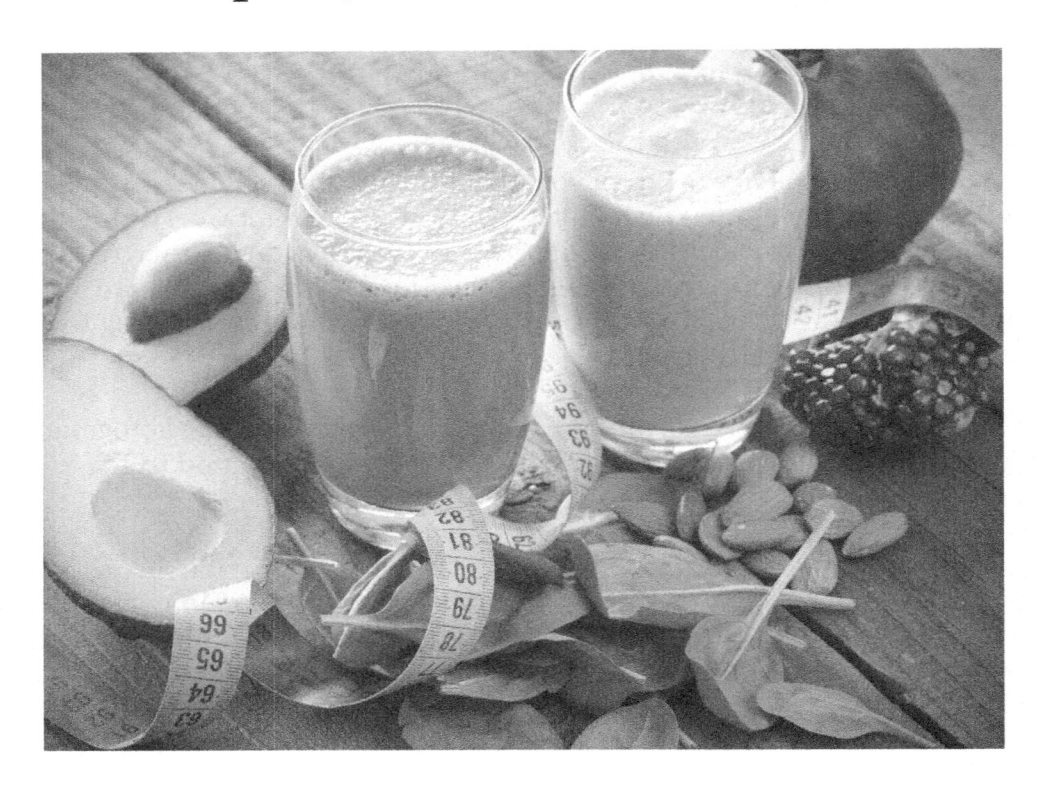

Smoothies & Beverages

Bulletproof Hot Chocolate

If you miss having hot chocolate, fear not - this is a vegan keto recipe for hot chocolate that you'll love!

Yields: 1 serving
Total prep & cooking time: 5 minutes
Nutrition Facts: Calories: 282 | Protein: 2.6 g | Net Carbohydrates: 8.2 g | Fat: 30.4 g

What to use:

- Unsweetened non-dairy milk (.5 cup)
- Hot water (not scalding) (.5 cup)
- Coconut oil (2 tablespoons)
- Cocoa powder - unsweetened (2 tablespoons)
- Your preferred liquid sweetener (1 to 2 tablespoons)
- Vanilla extract (0.25 teaspoon)

What to do:

1. Toss each of the fixings into your blender - blend till they become incorporated and creamy.
2. Serve the resulting hot chocolate and enjoy!

Healthy Green Smoothie

This super healthy smoothie makes for a great breakfast or a nice snack! It's packed with fiber and is suitable for a wide variety of diets. You can modify this with various additions, including protein powder, chia seeds, turmeric, or anything else that you think might be good!

Yields: 1 serving
Total prep & cooking time: 5 minutes
Nutrition Facts: Calories: 341 | Protein: 5.6 g | Fat: 24.7 g| Net Carbohydrates: 4.1 g

What to use:

- Baby spinach (.66 cup)
- Avocado (0.5 of a whole)
- Coconut oil (1 scoop, melted)
- Your preferred liquid sweetener (1 tablespoon)
- Vanilla extract (1 teaspoon)
- Matcha powder (.5 teaspoon)
- Water (.66 cup)
- Your preferred non-dairy milk (.5 cup)
- Ice cubes (5 total)

What to do:

1. Toss each of the fixings into your blender - mix till they are combined well.
2. That's all that is required for this recipe!
3. Serve and enjoy.

Tasty Turmeric Milkshake

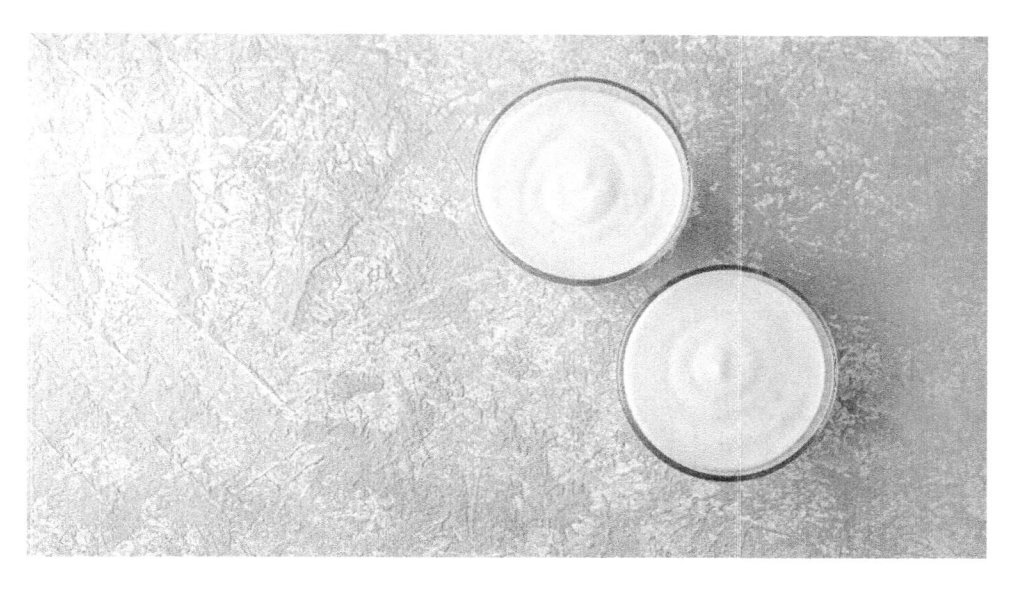

You'll remain satisfied and feel full for hours which makes this shake an excellent choice for a breakfast drink. It's not too sweet and is packed with flavor.

Yields: 1 serving
Total prep & cooking time: 5 minutes
Nutrition Facts: Calories: 351 |Protein: 1.6 g | Fat: 35 g| Net Carbohydrates: 7 g

What to use:

- Non-dairy milk (1.5 cups)
- Coconut oil (2 tablespoons, melted)
- Ground ginger (0.5 teaspoon, or 0.5 inches of peeled ginger root, finely grated)
- Vanilla (.25 teaspoon)
- Cinnamon (.25 teaspoon)
- Turmeric powder (.75 teaspoon)
- Salt (a pinch)
- Your preferred granulated sweetener (1 teaspoon, or more if you'd like it sweeter)
- Ice cubes (2 total)

What to do:

1. Measure and toss each of the ingredients in your blender. Mix thoroughly till all of the ingredients are well combined.
2. Pour the resulting milkshake into your glass and sprinkle some extra cinnamon and turmeric on the top of it.
3. Drink the milkshake and enjoy it!

Thai Iced Tea

Thai iced tea is a delectable combination of milk, tea, and sweetener. It's wonderfully delicious and really easy to make.

Yields: 4 servings
Total prep & cooking time: 15 minutes
Nutrition Facts: Calories: 65 | Protein: -0- g | Net Carbs: 1 g | Fat: 7 g

What to use:

- Water (4 cups)
- Black tea bags (4 regular-sized bags)
- Cardamom pods (5 total, crushed)
- Star anise pods (3 total)
- Cloves (2 whole)
- Water (room temperature is fine) (3 cups)
- Cinnamon (0.5 to 1 teaspoon)
- Full-fat coconut milk (1 can)
- MCT oil (2 tablespoons)
- Vanilla extract (0.25 teaspoon)
- Your preferred sweetener (0.25 teaspoon)
- Ice (for serving)

What to do:

1. Boil the water in a saucepan on a stovetop - set using a high-temperature setting. Once the water is boiling, transfer the pan to a cool burner.
2. Put the tea bags, cardamom, star anise, cloves, and cinnamon into the pot and let all of this steep for about 10 minutes.
3. While the tea is steeping, put the coconut milk, vanilla extract, and MCT oil into the blender - mix till it's thoroughly combined.
4. Strain the ingredients out of the water. Pour in three cups of room temperature water into the cooking pot.
5. Put ice in your glasses. Fill each glass about half full with tea (and no more than ¾ full) with tea.
6. Fill the remainder of the glass with the MCT oil cream.
7. Stir, serve, and enjoy!

Vegan Bulletproof Coffee

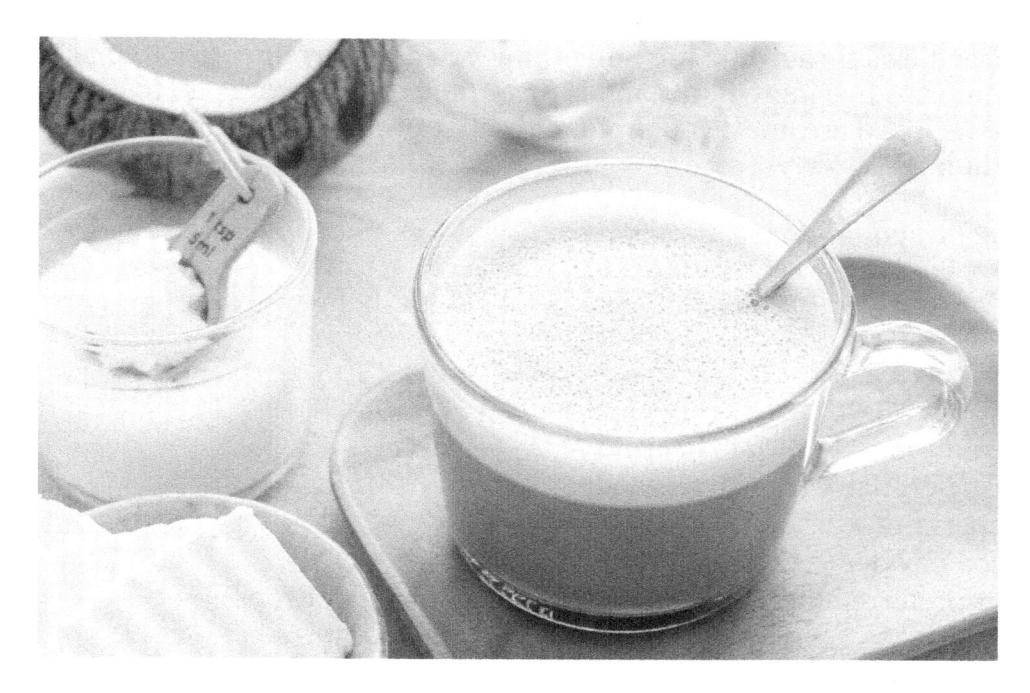

Bulletproof coffee is a great way to extend your overnight fast but not feel hungry, thanks to the coconut oil in the drink.

Yields: 1 cup
Total prep & cooking time: 5 minutes
Nutrition Facts: Calories: 123 | Protein: 0 g | Net Carbs: 0 g | Fat: 14 g

What to use:

- Your preferred coffee (hot) (1 cup)
- Coconut oil (1 tablespoon)
- Your preferred non-dairy milk (2 tablespoons to 0.25 cup)
- Optional: your preferred liquid sweetener (5 drops)

What to do:

1. Pour your favorite freshly brewed coffee into a blender.
2. Mix in the remainder of the fixings.
3. Serve the drink in a mug to your liking.

Coffee Creamer - Mint Chocolate

While this isn't exactly a drink, it is something you add to your coffee to make it even tastier. It only has five ingredients and is incredibly easy. It works up to a thick texture, almost like whipped cream. If you prefer a thinner product, you can add some more non-dairy milk.

Yields: 24 tablespoon-sized servings
Total prep & cooking time: 5 minutes
Nutrition Facts: Calories: 20 | Protein: -0- g | Net Carbohydrates: -0- g | Fat: 2 g

What to use:

- Coconut milk - full-fat (1 cup)
- Milk (non-dairy & unsweetened) (1.5 cup)
- Peppermint extract (0.25 teaspoon)
- Cocoa powder (2 tablespoons)
- Your preferred liquid sweetener (we used stevia) (5 drops)

What to do:

1. Measure and add each of the ingredients into your blender and mix till it's combined thoroughly.
2. That's all you need to do! Store the resulting creamer in the fridge and use it in your morning coffee for a delicious, minty treat.

Breakfast Goodies

Apple Pie Pancakes

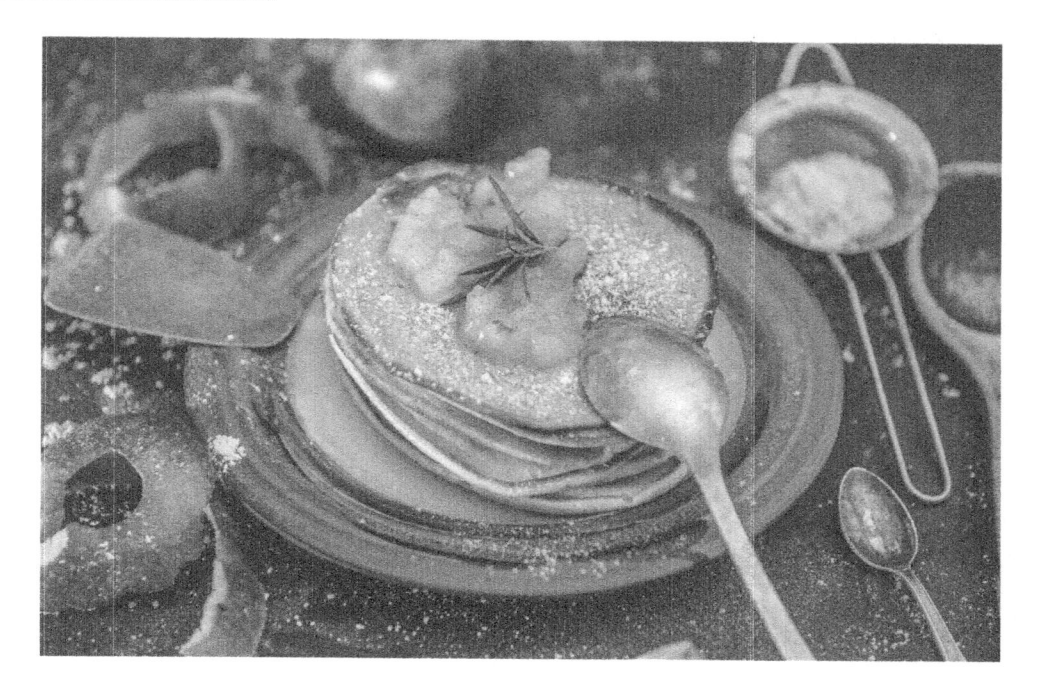

Yields: 3 servings
Total prep & cooking time: 7 minutes
Nutrition Facts: Calories: 125 | Protein: 7 g | Net Carbs: 3.5 g | Fat: 7 g

What to use:

- Coconut flour (2 tablespoons)
- Almond flour (.5 cup)
- Baking powder (1 tablespoon)
- Non-dairy milk (0.25 cup)
- Unsweetened applesauce (.5 cup)
- Monk fruit/another keto sweetener (1 tablespoon)
- Apple cider vinegar (1 tablespoon)
- Apple pie spice (1 teaspoon)

What to do:

1. The spices are to be mixed into the applesauce and combined well.
2. Toss each of the fixings into your blender. Mix it using the high-speed setting till it's creamy smooth.
3. Let the batter rest for at least five minutes, preferably a little more.

4. Place a pan over a stove burner heated to medium and give the pan time to heat. Spray with cooking spray to prevent sticking. Use a (0.25 cup) measuring cup and scoop the pancake batter into the heated pan.
5. Prepare the pancake for 1 or 2 minutes, then turn it over and continue cooking till it is nicely browned and thoroughly cooked (1-2 min.).
6. Continue cooking in this way until you have used all of the batter.

Avocado Smoothie with Matcha

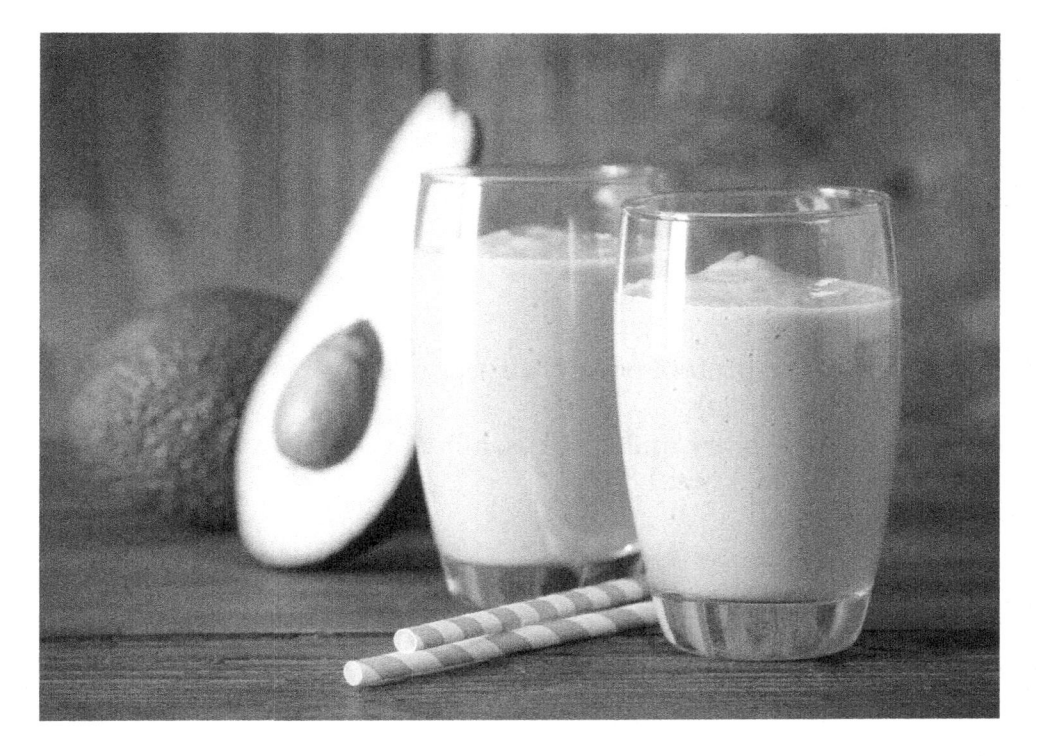

Avocados are among the best foods to eat on the keto diet because they're so high in healthy fats. This smoothie combines the deliciousness of avocados matcha and some citrusy flavors to make a fantastic smoothie that you're sure to love.

Yields: 1 serving
Total prep & cooking time: 5 minutes
Nutrition Facts: Calories: 229 | Protein: 14.1 g | Fat: 16.7 g | Net Carbohydrates: 4.4 g

What to use:

- Avocado (1 whole)
- Lime (1 whole, juice & rind)
- Lemon (1 whole, juice and rind)
- Matcha powder (1 tablespoon)
- Your preferred non-dairy milk (1 cup)
- Vanilla extract (1 teaspoon)
- (Optional) liquid sweetener of your choice and vanilla protein powder (1 scoop)

What to do:

1. Mix each of the fixings in your blender - blending well till it becomes an acceptable smoothie consistency.
2. Serve the resulting smoothie in a glass and enjoy!

Avocado Protein Smoothie

Another delicious, easy breakfast smoothie! This smoothie is low-carb and has a nice amount of fat and protein to keep you feeling full till lunch.

Yields: 2 servings
Total prep & cooking time: 3 minutes
Nutrition Facts: Calories: 634 | Protein: 35 g | Net Carbs: 11 g | Fat: 53.7 g

What to use:

- Your favorite Vegan protein powder (2 scoops)
- Avocado (0.5 of a whole)
- Your preferred non-dairy milk (3 cups, adjust the amount depending on the desired smoothie thickness)
- Ice (1 cup)
- Coconut oil (4 tablespoons)
- Hemp hearts (3 tablespoons)
- Ground flaxseed (2 tablespoons)
- Your preferred liquid sweetener (a few drops)

What to do:

1. Add each of the fixings in your blender - mix them till they become well combined.
2. That's all there is to do for this smoothie! Serve in your favorite glasses and enjoy.

Cinnamon Roll Muffins

Yields: 20 muffins
Total prep & cooking time: 20 minutes
Nutrition facts: Calories: 112 | Protein: 5 g | Fat: 9 g | Net Carbohydrates: 3 g

What to use:

The Muffin:
- Almond flour (.5 cup)
- Baking powder (1 teaspoon)
- Vegan protein powder (2 scoops)
- Cinnamon (1 tablespoon)
- Unsweetened applesauce (.5 cup)
- Preferred nut butter (.5 cup)
- Coconut oil (0.5 cup)

The Glaze:

- Non-dairy milk of your choice .5 cup)
- Stevia powder (1 tablespoon)
- Lemon juice (2 teaspoons)
- Coconut butter (0.25 cup)

Also Needed:

- Paper liners
- 12-count muffin tin

What to do:

1. Ensure that your oven is allowed time to preheat to 350° Fahrenheit/177° Celsius.
2. Put liners into the wells of the muffin tin and set them to the side for later use.
3. Mix the dry fixings in a big mixing container. The wet fixings should be added to these dry ingredients and combined thoroughly and completely.
4. Evenly distribute the batter into the cups of the prepared muffin tins. Bake the filled muffin tin for nearly 15 minutes.
5. Check the doneness of the muffins with a toothpick inserted into the muffin. It will be done when the toothpick comes cleanly out of the muffin. Leave the muffins in the pan to cool for a few moments, and then remove them to a wire rack so that they can cool down completely.
6. Combine the glaze fixings in a mixing container until they are combined well and thoroughly. Drizzle this over the cooled muffins and allow plenty of time for the glaze to set.

Crumbly Blueberry Bars

Yields: 8 bars
Total prep & cooking time: 35 minutes
Nutrition Facts: Calories: 315 | Protein: 10 g | Net Carbs: 6 g | Fat: 18 g

What to use:

Bars:

- Blanched almond flour (1 cup)
- Baking soda (.5 teaspoon)
- Coconut (0.75 cup - unsweetened and shredded)
- Keto maple syrup (0.25 cup)
- Coconut oil (.5 cup melted)
- Blueberries (1 cup)
- Vegan blueberry jam (.5 cup)
- Unsweetened applesauce (0.25 to 0.5 cup)

Crumb topping:

- Coconut flour (0.5 tablespoon)
- Stevia powder (2 tablespoons)
- Blanched almond flour (.5 cup)
- Vanilla extract (.5 teaspoon)
- Coconut oil (2 tablespoons, melted)
- Keto maple syrup (2 tablespoons)

What to do:

1. Ensure enough time for your oven to preheat to 350° Fahrenheit/177° Celsius.
2. Carefully line an 8" baking pan with parchment paper, ensuring complete coverage.
3. In your large mixing bowl, add all of your dry ingredients to combine (Note: ¼ of a cup of the applesauce, the syrup, and the coconut oil should be mixed in another mixing container).
4. Combine the dry ingredients with the wet ingredients in the wet ingredients bowl and combine by stirring. If the mixture is thicker than it should be, add the remaining 0.25 cup of the applesauce and stir more.
5. Retrieve the parchment-lined pan and press the bar mixture into the pan. Be sure that the mixture is spread evenly. Smooth the vegan blueberry jam over the top of the bar mixture, then distribute the blueberries over the jam's top.

6. Create the crumb topping. The dry ingredients for the crumb topping should be added to a small bowl and combined.
7. Using a different mixing container, whisk the vanilla extract with the keto maple syrup and coconut oil. Mix in the dry fixings into the wet ingredients - stir till the mixture's consistency is similar to tiny crumbles.
8. Sprinkle the crumbled topping over the bar mixture in the pan and pop it into the oven to bake till the topping is beginning to turn a lovely golden color (25 min.).
9. Leave it in the pan until the bars are cooled down completely, and then slice the mixture into bar shapes.

Crust-Free Mini Quiche

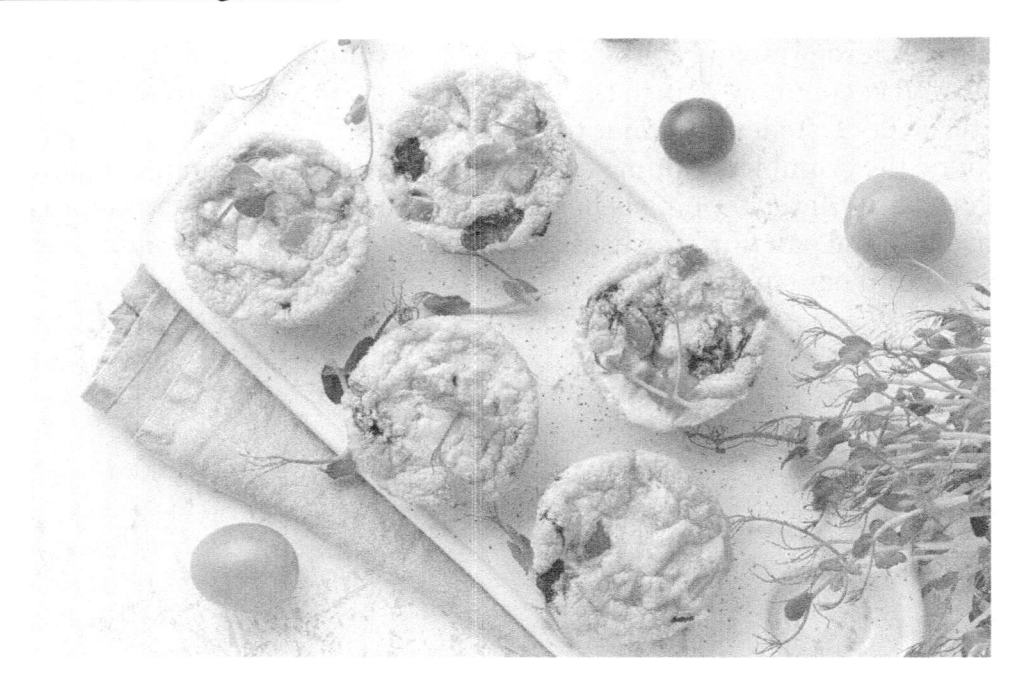

Yields: 12 mini quiche portions
Total prep & cooking time: 45 minutes
Nutrition Facts: Calories: 163 | Protein: 11 g | Fat: 9.9 g | Net Carbohydrates: 9.6 g

What to use:

- Water, warm (1 cup)
- Extra-firm tofu (1 block)
- Ground flax seeds (.5 cup)
- Hemp seeds (.5 cup)
- Baking powder (1 teaspoon)
- Nutritional yeast (.5 cup)
- Salt (1 teaspoon)
- Almond flour (.5 cup)
- Sun-dried tomatoes (.25 cup, chopped finely)
- Italian seasoning (2 teaspoons)
- Chia seeds (.25 cup)

What to do:

1. Thoroughly warm the oven before baking time till it reaches 350° Fahrenheit or 177° Celsius.

2. Using a baking spray to prepare the muffin tin, spray each muffin cup and set the pan to the side.
3. Mix the warm water and the flaxseed and set aside for ten minutes to allow the flaxseed to gel.
4. Prepare the tofu by pressing and draining the tofu water from the block. Make the tofu into small pieces by crumbling or cutting it into the large bowl.
5. Combine the remaining ingredients in the mixing container with the tofu. Combine the gelled flaxseed mixture and thoroughly mix.
6. Spoon the resulting mixture evenly into the muffin tin you have prepared.
7. Bake the muffin mixture in the tin for about 35 minutes, and then cool for 10 minutes in the tin before removing them from the muffin tin.
8. Note: If you desire a smoother texture for the quiche, pulse the fixings in a food processor.

Low-Carb Maple "Oatmeal"

Yields: 4 servings
Total prep & cooking time: 25 minutes
Nutrition Facts: Calories: 374 | Protein: 9.25 g | Net Carbs: 12.37 g | Fat: 34.59 g

What to use:

- Sunflower seeds (0.6 cups)
- Walnuts and pecans (.5 cup of each)
- Chia seeds (4 tablespoons)
- Shredded coconut or coconut flakes (2.5 tablespoons)
- Unsweetened and unflavored non-dairy milk (4.3 cups)
- Stevia powder (0.375 teaspoons)
- Cinnamon .5 teaspoon)

What to do:

1. Put walnuts, sunflower seeds, and pecans into your high-powered food processor - repeatedly pulse till all sunflower seeds, walnuts, and pecans are chopped thoroughly.
2. Toss each of the fixings into a pot. Set the stove's heat to a low-temperature setting and simmer (20-30 min.). Stir the pot's contents occasionally so that the chopped seeds and ingredients do not stick to the bottom of the pot. Cook this mixture until the chia seeds have soaked up almost all of the liquid in the pot.
3. Once your "oatmeal" mixture is thickened, take it off of the heated burner and serve the oatmeal mixture in a bowl. The oatmeal mixture tastes best when it is hot and fresh out of the pot. The oatmeal can be cooled and stored in the fridge for eating the next day, but be sure to heat it thoroughly before eating so that you enjoy the full flavor.
4. Serve the oatmeal with fresh fruit or a few chopped nuts over the top.

Overnight Vanilla "Oatmeal"

Yields: 1 serving
Total prep & cooking time: 5 minutes
Nutrition Facts: Calories: 408 | Protein: 15.3 g | Fat: 34.7 g | Net Carbohydrates: 9.1 g

What to use:

- Hemp seeds (or flax seeds) (.5 cup)
- Chia seeds (1 tablespoon)
- Full-fat non-dairy milk (.66 cup)
- Liquid stevia (3 to 4 drops)
- Vanilla extract (.5 teaspoon)
- Salt (a pinch)

What to do:

1. All ingredients are to be placed into a container with a lid. Stir these ingredients until they are combined. Place the lid on the container and set the container into the refrigerator overnight (minimum of 8 hrs.).
2. After 8 hours, remove the mixture from the fridge. Place more non-dairy milk into the mixture and stir until the oatmeal arrives at your preferred consistency.
3. This dish can be served plain or with almonds and fruit sprinkled over the top.

Tasty Tofu Scramble

Yields: 4 servings
Total preparation & cooking time: 18-20 minutes
Nutritional Facts: Calories: 141 | Protein: 12 g | Net Carbs: 8g | Fat: 8 g

What to use:

- Extra-firm tofu (1 block)
- Ground turmeric (2 teaspoons)
- Black pepper (0.25 teaspoon)
- Salt (.5 teaspoon)
- Avocado oil (1.5 tablespoons)
- Fresh chives for serving (optional, just a pinch)

What to do:

1. Drain and press the tofu.
2. Your pressed tofu shall be crumbled, chopped, or broken up into minuscule pieces.
3. Warm a pan on the stovetop using a medium-temperature setting to heat the oil.
4. Place the tofu into this heated pan over the burner and allow the tofu to cook for nearly 7 minutes.
5. If you desire softer scrambled tofu, you can use non-dairy milk (0.25 cup) and toss it into the tofu mixture in the pan. Allow it to cook for another moment. This step is purely up to you and is not necessary.
6. Scramble is most delicious while warm and fresh from the stovetop pan.

Chapter 6: Lunch Favorites

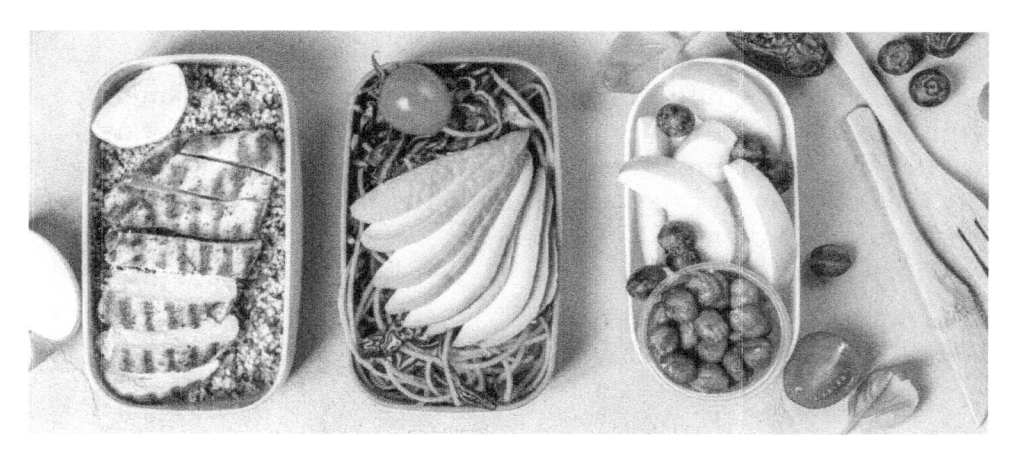

Salad Option

Arugula Salad with Cherry Tomatoes

This salad is so flavorful! It's loaded with arugula, avocado, and cherry tomatoes. It's also topped with a tasty balsamic vinaigrette. It makes a great side dish, but it also works as a delicious lunch.

Yields: 4 servings
Total prep & cooking time: 15 minutes
Nutrition Facts: Calories: 269 | Protein: 3 g | Net Carbs: 1 g | Fat: 17 g

What to use:

For the salad:

- Red & Yellow cherry tomatoes (1 pint of each, cut into halves)
- Avocados (2 large)
- Arugula (5 ounces, roughly chopped)
- Fresh basil leaves (6 leaves, sliced thinly)
- Red onion (.25 cup - diced)

For the vinaigrette:

- Olive oil (1 tablespoon)
- Italian seasoning (.5 teaspoon)
- Garlic (1 clove, minced)
- Lemon juice (1 tablespoon)
- Balsamic vinegar (2 tablespoons)
- Keto-friendly maple-flavored syrup - ex. Lakanto (1 tablespoon)

- Black pepper and salt (0.25 teaspoon, or as desired)

What to do:

1. Toss the salad fixings into a big mixing container - gently tossing them till they are combined.
2. Whisk the vinaigrette ingredients together until thoroughly combined.
3. Empty the dressing over the salad - gently tossing it to be sure the dressing is coating every ingredient.
4. Serve with a garnish of basil.

Grab & Go Jar Salad

Yields: 1 serving
Total prep & cooking time: 5-6 minutes
Nutrition Facts: Calories: 215 | Protein: 8 g | Net Carbs: 4 g | Fat: 19 g

What to use:

- Black pepper & salt (as desired)
- Keto-friendly mayonnaise (4 tablespoons)
- Scallion (half of 1)
- Cucumber (.25 ounce)
- Red bell pepper (.25 ounce)
- Cherry tomatoes (.25 ounce)
- Leafy greens (.25 ounce)
- Seasoned tempeh (4 ounces)

What to do:

1. Chop or shred the vegetables as desired.
2. Layer in the dark leafy greens first, followed by the onions, tomato, bell peppers, avocado, and shredded carrot.
3. Top with the tempeh, or use the same amount of another high-protein option to mix things up in later weeks.
4. Top with keto-vegan mayonnaise before serving.

Greek Chopped Salad

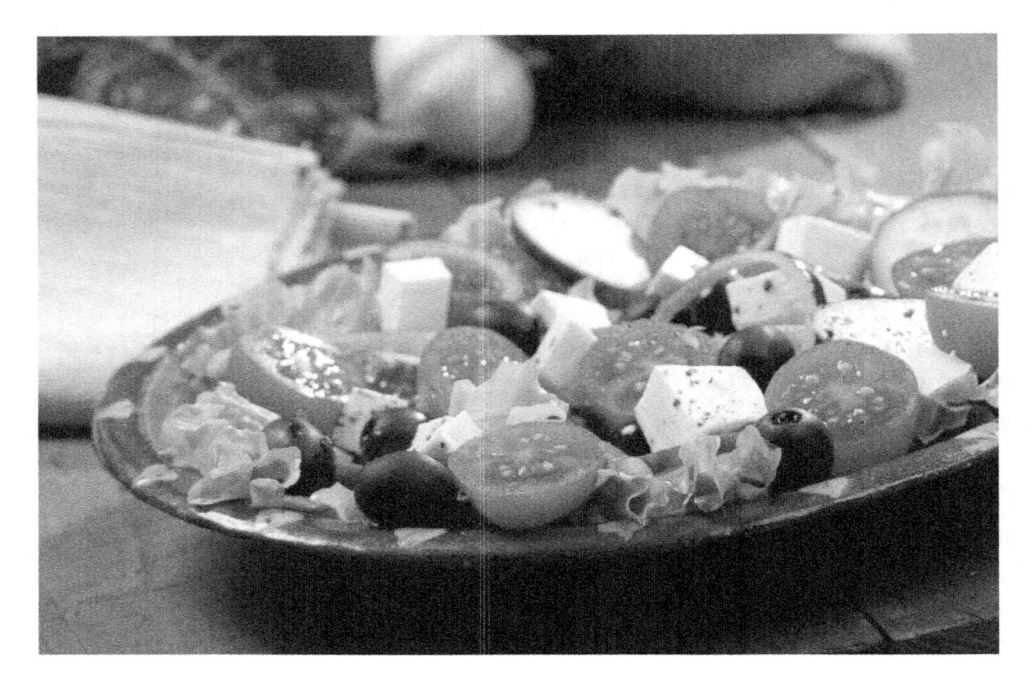

Yields: 2 servings
Total prep & cooking time: 5 minutes
Nutrition Facts: Calories: 202 | Protein: 4 g | Net Carbs: 2 g | Fat: 19 g

What to use:

- Chopped romaine (2 cups)
- Halved grape tomatoes (.5 cup)
- Kalamata black olives (.25 cup)
- Crumbled feta cheese (.25 cup)
- Olive oil (1 tablespoon)
- Vinaigrette dressing (2 tablespoons)
- Black pepper & Pink salt (as desired)

What to do:

1. Put the salad together using lettuce as a base.
2. Spritz it using a drizzle of oil and vinegar.
3. Serve in two salad dishes.

Kale Salad

Yields: 4 servings
Total prep & cooking time: 8-10 minutes
Nutrition Facts: Calories: 80 | Protein: 4 g | Net Carbs: 3 g | Fat: 6 g

What to use:

- Salt (.5 teaspoon)
- Olive oil (1 tablespoon)
- Kale (1 bunch)
- Lemon juice (1 tablespoon)
- Parmesan cheese (.33 cup)

What to do:

1. Remove the ribs from the kale and slice into ¼-inch strips.
2. Combine with the salt and oil, toss till softened (3 min.).
3. Toss the cheese, juice, and kale. Serve.

Soup

Avocado Mint Chilled Soup

Yields: 2 servings
Preparation and cook time: 18-20 minutes
Nutrition Facts: Calories: 280 | Protein: 4 g | Net Carbs: 4 g | Fat: 26 g

What to use:

- Romaine lettuce (2 leaves)
- Ripened avocado (1 medium)
- Coconut milk (1 cup)
- Lime juice (1 tablespoon)
- Fresh mint (20 leaves)
- Salt (as desired)

What to do:

1. Combine all of the fixings into a blender and mix well. You want it thick but not puree-like.
2. Chill in the refrigerator for five to ten minutes before serving.

Carrot Onion & Beef Soup - Instant Pot

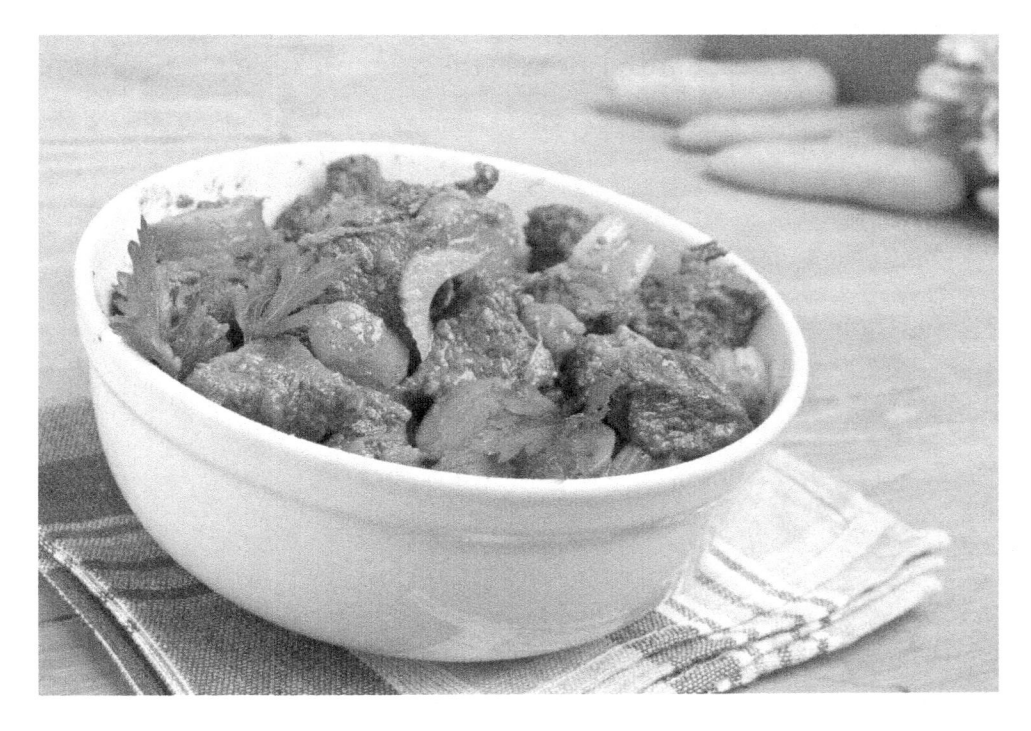

Yields: 4 servings
Total prep & cooking time: minutes
Nutrition Facts: Calories: 328 | Protein: 25 g | Net Carbs: 3 g | Fat: 65 g

What to use:

- Beef stew meat (2 lb./910 g)
- Pepper & Salt (as desired)
- Cooking oil (2 tbsp.)
- Tomato paste (1 tbsp.)
- Garlic cloves (4)
- Sliced onion (1)
- Sliced carrots (4 peeled)
- Beef broth (3 cups)
- Bay leaves (2)
- Thyme sprigs (6)
- Water (1 cup)

What to do:

1. Sprinkle the salt and pepper over the chopped beef.
2. Heat the Instant Pot using the sauté mode. Pour in the oil and add the beef. Saute it for four to five minutes until browned.

3. Chop and stir in the onions, garlic, and carrots. Simmer them for two minutes and toss in the bay leaves, thyme, broth, and tomato paste. Stir well.
4. Secure the lid and set the time for 30 minutes – manual setting.
5. When the timer buzzes, natural-release the pressure for eight to ten minutes and open the lid.
6. Season and serve it warm.

Chicken "Zoodle" Soup

Yields: 2 servings
Preparation and cook time: 18-25 minutes
Nutrition Facts: Calories: 310 | Protein: 34 g | Net Carbs: 4 g | Fat: 16 g

What to use:

- Chicken breast (1)
- Avocado oil (2 tablespoons)
- Green onion (1)
- Celery stalk (1)
- Chicken broth (3 cups)
- Cilantro (.25 cup)
- Salt (as desired)
- Zucchini (1)

What to do:

1. Chop or dice the breast of the chicken. Pour the oil into a saucepan and cook the chicken until done.
2. Pour in the broth and simmer.
3. Chop the celery and green onions and toss them into the pan. Simmer for 3-4 more minutes.
4. Chop the cilantro and prepare the zucchini noodles. Use a spiralizer or potato peeler to make the 'noodles.' (Remove the peel.) Add to the pot.
5. Simmer for a few more minutes and season to your liking.
6. Store in a glass container in the fridge. It will remain tasty for two to three days.

Superfood Soup

This soup contains a lot of micronutrients, which makes it extremely healthy. More importantly, it's also very tasty. It's packed with delicious, healthy vegetables, is high in antioxidants, and contains an excellent amount of vitamins and minerals.

Yields: 6 servings
Total prep & cooking time: 20 minutes
Nutritional Facts: Calories: 393 | Fat: 37.6 g | Protein: 4.9 g | Net Carbs: 6.8 g

What to use:

- Cauliflower (1 whole head)
- Medium onion (1 whole)
- Garlic cloves (2)
- Bay leaf (1 whole leaf - crumbled)
- Watercress (.66 cup)
- Fresh spinach (1 cup)
- Vegetable broth (4 cups)
- Coconut milk (1 cup)
- Coconut oil (0.25 cup - melted)
- Black pepper (as desired)
- Salt (1 teaspoon)

What to do:

1. Warm the oil in a pot on the stovetop using a med-high temperature setting.
2. Mince and toss in the onion and garlic - sautéing till they're lightly browned.
3. Place the cauliflower florets into the pot - cook for about five minutes. Stir occasionally. Mix in the watercress and spinach. Simmer till the spinach is wilted.
4. Add the vegetable stock. Wait for the mixture to boil. Cook till the cauliflower is tender but still a little crispy. Add the coconut milk, pepper, salt, and any desired spices.
5. Remove from heat and use an immersion blender until the soup is creamy.
6. Serve right away! This soup does keep well in the fridge for no more than five days. It freezes well also.

Warm Vegan Walnut Chili

Just as filling as chili with meat, but vegan-friendly! This walnut chili is warm and comforting, low-carb and high-protein.

Yields: 4 to 6 servings
Total prep & cooking time: 41 minutes
Nutrition Facts: Calories: 353| Protein: 13 g | Net Carbs: 18 g | Fat: 28 g

What to use:

- Celery (5 whole stalks, diced)
- Garlic cloves (2 whole, minced)
- Cinnamon (1.5 teaspoons)
- Chili powder (2 teaspoons)
- Paprika (1.5 teaspoons)
- Bell peppers (2 diced)
- Chipotle peppers (preferably chipotle in adobo) (2 whole, diced)
- Mushrooms (8 ounces)
- Tomato paste (1.5 tablespoons)
- Diced tomatoes (1 15 ounce can)
- Ground cumin (4 teaspoons)
- Coconut milk (.5 cup)
- Water (3 cups)
- Olive oil (2 tablespoons)
- Unsweetened cocoa powder (1 tablespoon)
- Vegan meat substitute (2.5 cups, crumbled)
- Raw walnuts (1 cup, chopped finely)
- Black pepper & salt (as desired)

Serve with:

- Avocado (2 whole, sliced)
- Cilantro leaves (2 tablespoons, chopped)
- Radishes (2 tablespoons, sliced)

What to do:

1. Prepare a Dutch oven on a stove burner - heated using the medium-temperature setting to warm the oil. Toss in the celery and sauté it for about four minutes.
2. Mix in the paprika, cumin, chili powder, cinnamon, and garlic. Stir and sauté the mixture until it begins to smell very nice (about another two minutes).
3. Add the mushrooms, zucchini, and bell peppers. Cook in the pan for five more minutes.

4. Mix in the tomato paste, water, tomatoes, coconut milk, chipotle, vegan meat, cocoa powder, and walnuts.
5. Reduce the temperature setting to med-low. Simmer till the vegetables are soft and the chili has become thick (20 min.).
6. Serve the chili with radishes, cilantro, and avocado with a shake of pepper and salt before serving.

Pasta Options

Asian BBQ Meatball Noodles Bowl

Yields: 4 servings
Total prep & cooking time: minutes
Nutrition Facts: Calories: 318 | Protein: 24 g | Net Carbs: 11 g | Fat: 20 g

What to use:

The BBQ Sauce:

- Sesame oil (1 tbsp.)
- Tamari (4 tbsp.)
- Rice wine vinegar (.25 cup)
- Granulated swerve (.25 cup)
- Sriracha (3 tbsp.)
- Fresh ginger (1 tbsp.)
- Clove of garlic (1)

The Meatballs:

- Ground chicken or turkey (1 pound)
- Shiitake mushrooms (.25 cup/20 g)
- Fresh cilantro (.25 cup)
- Green onions (2)
- Garlic cloves (2)
- Tamari (1 tbsp.)
- Fish sauce (1 teaspoon)
- Salt (.5 teaspoon)
- Red pepper flakes (.5 teaspoon)
- Sesame oil (2 tablespoons)

Other Fixings:

- Snow peas (8 ounces)
- Shirataki/Miracle noodles (2 packages)

What to do:

1. Mince the mushrooms, onions, ginger, and garlic.
2. Combine all of the meatball fixings (omitting the oil). Roll into 16 balls.
3. Whisk the sauce fixings and noodles. Set both aside for now.
4. Meanwhile, warm the oil in the skillet and add the meatballs - single layered.
5. Sear on each side and remove from the heat (2-3 min.).

6. Add the peas to the skillet to simmer for one minute until it starts to wilt.
7. Arrange the meatballs in the mixture and stir.
8. Simmer with a lid on the pot for about three minutes.

Baked Zucchini Noodles With Feta

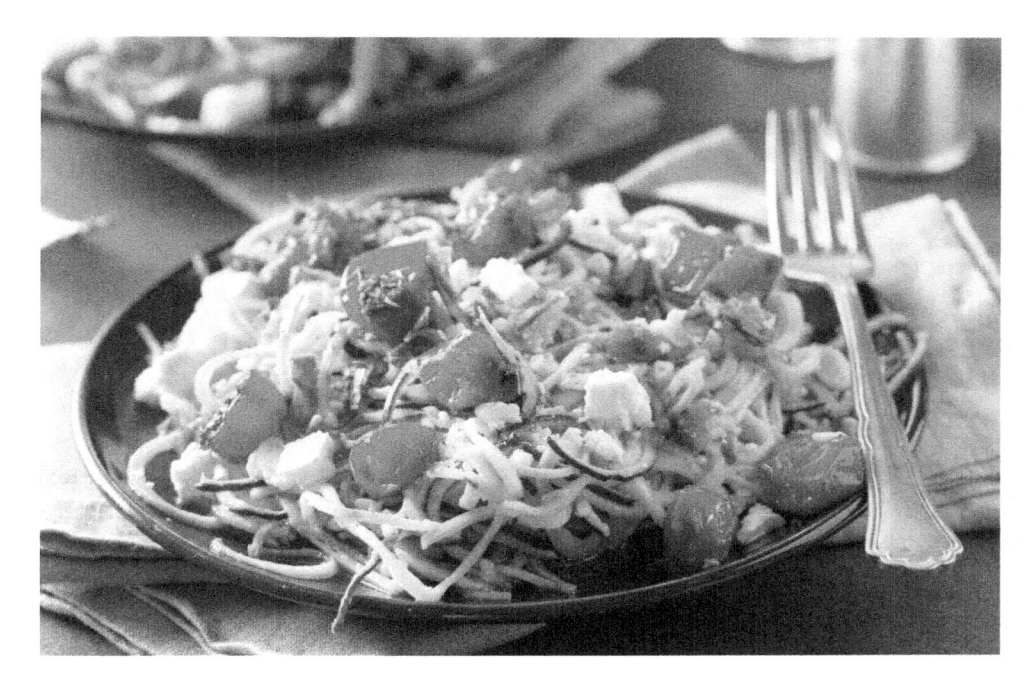

Yields: 3 servings
Total prep & cooking time: 25 minutes
Nutrition Facts: Calories: 105| Protein: 4 g | Net Carbs: 5 g | Fat: 8 g

What to use:

- Quartered plum tomato (1)
- Spiralized zucchini (2)
- Feta cheese (8 cubes)
- Pepper and salt (1 teaspoon of each)
- Olive oil (1 tablespoon)

What to do:

1. Lightly grease a roasting pan with a spritz of oil.
2. Set the oven temperature to reach 375° Fahrenheit/191° Celsius.
3. Slice the noodles with a spiralizer and add to the prepared pan with olive oil and tomatoes. Sprinkle it with pepper and salt.
4. Bake for 10 to 15 minutes. Transfer the pan from the oven and add the cheese cubes, tossing to combine. Serve.

Delicious Marinara Zoodles

Yields: 4 servings
Total prep & cooking time: 35-40 minutes
Nutrition Facts: Calories: 179| Protein: 7 g | Net Carbs: 5 g | Fat: 19 g

What to use:

- Olive oil (2 tablespoons)
- Garlic cloves (6)
- White onions (.5 cup)
- Tomatoes (14-ounce can)
- Tomato paste (2 tablespoons)
- Basil leaves (.5 cup - loosely packed)
- Coarse salt (1.5 teaspoons)
- Black pepper (.25 teaspoon)
- Cayenne (1 pinch)
- Spiralized zucchinis (2 large)

What to do:

1. Pour the oil into the skillet before placing it on the stovetop (medium heat setting).
2. Mince the garlic cloves, onions, and tomatoes. Roughly chop the basil leaves. Use a veggie peeler, knife, or spiralizer to prepare the zucchini.
3. Toss in and sauté the onion for about five minutes before adding in the garlic. Cook for approximately one minute.
4. Mix in the salt, crushed red pepper flakes, pepper, salt, basil, tomato paste, and tomatoes. Combine thoroughly.
5. Simmer the sauce and lower the temperature setting to medium-low. Simmer for another 15 minutes or until the oil takes on a deep orange color, indicating the sauce is thickened and reduced. Season as desired.
6. Add in the zoodles and let them soften approximately two minutes before serving.

Fettuccine Chicken Alfredo

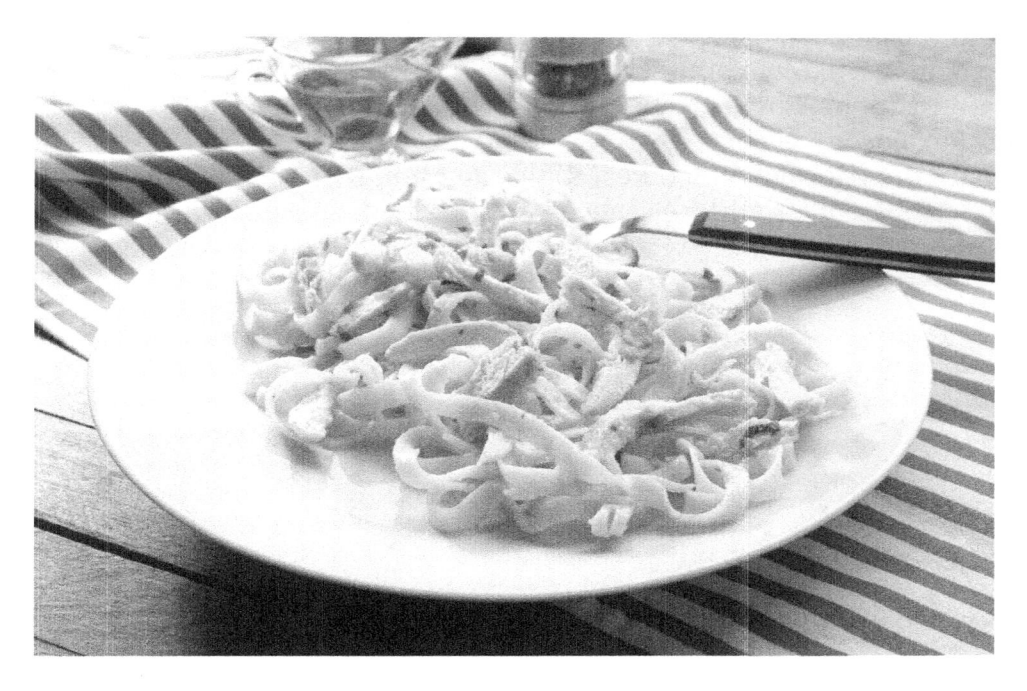

Yields: 2 servings
Total prep & cooking time: 40-45 minutes
Nutrition Facts: Calories: 585 | Protein: 25 g | Net Carbs: 1 g | Fat: 51 g

What to use:

- Butter (2 tablespoons)
- Minced garlic cloves (2)
- Dried basil (.5 teaspoon)
- Heavy cream (.5 cup)
- Grated parmesan (4 tablespoons)

The Chicken & Noodles:

- Chicken thighs - no bones or skin (2)
- Olive oil (1 tablespoon)
- Miracle Noodle - Fettuccini (1 bag)
- Salt and pepper (as desired)

What to do:

1. Prepare the sauce by adding the butter and cloves to a pan - sauté for two minutes.
2. Measure and add the cream into the skillet and simmer it for another two minutes.

3. Mix in one tablespoon of the parmesan at a time. Add the salt, pepper, and dried basil. Simmer using the low-temperature setting (3-5 min.).
4. Pound the chicken using a meat tenderizer hammer until it's ½-inch thick.
5. Warm oil in a skillet using the medium temperature setting.
6. Arrange the chicken in the pan to cook for about seven minutes per side. Shred and set aside.
7. Prepare the package of noodles. Rinse, and boil them in a pot of water (2 min.).
8. Fold in the noodles with the sauce and shredded chicken. Simmer them for two minutes and serve.

Healthy Edamame Kelp Noodles

Yields: 2 servings
Total prep & cooking time: 10 minutes
Nutrition Facts: Calories: 139 | Protein: 8 g | Net Carbs: 5 g | Fat: 9 g

What to use:

- Kelp noodles (1 package)
- Shelled edamame (.5 cup)
- Julienned carrots (.25 cup)
- Sliced mushrooms (.25 cup)
- Frozen spinach (1 cup)

The Sauce:

- Sesame oil (1 tablespoon)
- Tamari (2 tablespoons)
- Ground ginger (.5 teaspoon)
- Garlic powder (.5 teaspoon)
- Sriracha (.25 teaspoon)

What to do:

1. Soak the noodles in water. Drain in a colander when ready.
2. Use the medium setting and combine the sauce fixings in a saucepan. Add the veggies and warm.
3. Stir in the noodles and simmer for two to three minutes, stirring occasionally.

Peanut Red Curry Vegan Bowl - Thai-Inspired

Yields: 1 serving
Total prep & cooking time: 15-20 minutes
Nutrition Facts: Calories: 355 | Protein: 16 g | Net Carbs: 10 g | Fat: 23 g

What to use:

- Sesame oil (1 teaspoon)
- Shirataki noodles (8-ounce package)
- Unsweetened peanut butter (2 tablespoons)
- Low-sodium tamari (2 teaspoons)
- Thai red curry paste (2-3 teaspoons)
- Grated ginger (.25 teaspoon))
- Fresh edamame (.25 cup)
- Fresh lime juice (1 teaspoon)

Optional Garnishes Needed:

- Chopped peanuts
- Additional lime juice
- Red pepper flakes (1 pinch)

What to do:

1. Thoroughly rinse and drain the noodles and add to a frying pan using the medium-low temperature setting. Cook for a few minutes until the noodles are mostly dry.
2. Stir in the curry paste, tamari, peanut butter, sesame oil, grated ginger, and bell peppers. Stir until a sauce forms and everything is evenly coated.
3. Simmer for about three to five more minutes or until the peppers soften, and everything is heated.
4. Transfer the hot curry to a bowl and top with edamame and other desired toppings.

Zucchini Lasagna

This lasagna is easy and delicious and will fulfill your Italian food cravings without carbs or dairy.

Yields: 9 servings
Total preparation & cook time: 1 hr. & 20 min.
Nutritional Facts: Calories: 338 | Protein: 4.7 g | Fat: 34 g | Net Carbohydrates: 10 g

What to use:

- Zucchini (3 whole medium-sized)
- Extra-firm tofu (1 whole block, drained and pressed)
- Fresh basil (0.5 cup - packed & chopped)
- Nutritional yeast (2 tablespoons)
- Dried oregano (2 teaspoons)
- Water (0.25 to 0.5 cup)
- Lemon juice (2 tablespoons - freshly squeezed)
- Olive oil (1 tablespoon)
- Vegan parmesan cheese (0.25 cup)
- Black pepper (a pinch)
- Salt (1 teaspoon)
- Your favorite marinara sauce (1 jar)

What to do:

1. Ensure ample time to preheat your oven to 375° Fahrenheit/191° Celsius.
2. Slice the zucchini into long strips. Use a mandolin for thin, even slices, or carefully slice the zucchini with a sharp knife.
3. Put the tofu in a food processor - pulse to mix.
4. Load it with lemon juice, olive oil, basil, nutritional yeast, oregano, pepper, salt, water, and vegan parmesan cheese - blend these ingredients until they become a well-pureed paste.
5. Pour a cup of sauce into a 13-inch baking dish. Cover the base of the dish with zucchini slices on top of the sauce. Drop a couple of spoonfuls of the mixture from the blender over the zucchini and spread gently to cover the zucchini slices. Add another layer of marinara, more zucchini slices, and more "cheese" mixture.
6. Continue making layers until you run out of ingredients, finishing with two layers of zucchini slices and sauce.
7. Cover the baking dish with a layer of foil. Bake it in the preheated oven for about 45 minutes. Discard the foil - bake for an additional 15 minutes. The zucchini should become tender. Let the lasagna cool for about ten minutes before you slice it.
8. Top with more vegan parmesan cheese and fresh basil.
9. The lasagna is delicious for two days - freeze it for up to a month.

Zucchini Noodle Alfredo - Vegan-Friendly

It's not quite fettuccine alfredo, but close and not nearly as full of carbs. Use macadamia nuts to create the rich sauce and use it to top zucchini noodles for a delicious meal. You can also use this alfredo on spaghetti squash.

Yields: 4 servings
Total preparation & cooking time: 15-25 minutes
Nutrition Facts: Calories: 198 | Protein: 11 g | Fat: 16 g| Net Carbohydrates: 11.4 g

What to use:

- Roasted macadamia nuts (1 cup)
- Hot water (1 cup)
- Lemon (0.5 of a whole, for juice and zest)
- Garlic salt (.5 teaspoon)
- Nutritional yeast (.5 cup)
- Olive oil (4 tablespoons)
- Zucchini (4 whole, or buy zucchini noodles at the store)

To garnish:

- Chopped parsley
- Chopped macadamia nuts (0.25 cup)
- Freshly ground black pepper

What to do:

1. Put macadamia nuts and hot water into a food processor and allow to sit for five minutes. Mix in the lemon zest, nutritional yeast, garlic salt, and half of the olive oil. Blend these ingredients thoroughly until the mixture becomes a completely smooth consistency.
2. Spiralize the zucchini into a bowl. Alternatively, you can use zucchini noodles that you have bought from the store. If you do this, use this step to put your store-bought zucchini noodles into the bowl.
3. Warm a pan on the stovetop using the med-high temperature setting to warm the rest of the olive oil. Fold in the zucchini noodles. Cook for a few minutes until it becomes slightly wilted. Season the ingredients in the pan with more garlic salt.
4. Pour in the sauce and toss the noodles to coat. Cook until heated through, then serve, garnish, and enjoy!

Chapter 7: Keto Dinners

Poultry

Bruschetta Chicken

Yields: 4 servings
Total prep & cooking time: 60 minutes
Nutrition Facts: Calories: 480| Fat: 26 g | Protein: 52 g |Net Carbohydrates: 4 g

What to use:

- Olive oil (0.33 cup)
- Balsamic vinegar (2 tablespoons)
- Cloves of garlic (2 teaspoons - minced)
- Sea salt (.5 teaspoon)
- Black pepper (1 teaspoon)
- Sun-dried tomatoes in olive oil (.5 cup)
- Chicken breasts – quartered – boneless (2 pounds)
- Freshly chopped basil (2 tablespoons)

What to do:

1. Whisk the oil with the vinegar, garlic, pepper, and salt in a mixing container.
2. Fold in the tomatoes and basil.
3. Put the breasts in a freezer bag with the mixture for 30 minutes.
4. Add all of the fixings into the Instant Pot and secure the lid.
5. Select the poultry setting (9 min.). Natural-release the pressure for five minutes, quick-release, and serve.

Creamy Instant Pot Chicken

Yields: 4 Servings
Total preparation & cooking time: ½ hour
Nutrition Facts: Calories: 405| Fat: 31 g | Protein: 21 g |Net Carbs: 9 g

What to use - the Sauce:

- Garlic (6 cloves)
- Onion (1 chopped)
- Ginger (1 to 2-inch knot)
- Full-fat coconut milk (.5 cup)
- Powdered chicken broth base (1 tablespoon)
- Rotel canned tomato and chilis (10-ounce can)
- Ground turmeric (1 teaspoon)

What to use - the Chicken:

- Chopped celery (1.5 cups)
- Chopped Swiss chard (2 cups)
- Chicken thighs (1 pound)

What to use - the Finish:

- Full-fat coconut milk (.5 cup)

What to do:

1. Put the coconut milk, broth base, turmeric, garlic, onion, ginger, tomatoes, and chilis into a blender. Roughly puree the sauce and add to the Instant Pot.
2. Toss in the celery, chard, and chopped chicken.
3. Select the soup setting (5 min. under high-pressure). Natural release for ten minutes, and quick-release the rest.
4. Pour in the remainder of the coconut milk, stir, and enjoy.

French Garlic Chicken

Yields: 4 Portions
Total preparation & cooking time: ½ hour
Nutrition Facts: Calories: 429| Fat: 37 g | Protein: 19 g |Net Carbohydrates: 4 g

What to use - the Marinade:

- Olive oil (2 tablespoons)
- Prepared Dijon mustard (1 tablespoon)
- Cider vinegar (1 tablespoon)
- Minced garlic (1 tablespoon)
- Herbes de Provence (2 teaspoons)
- Black pepper & salt (1 teaspoon of each)
- Chicken thighs – no bones or skin (1 pound)

What to use:

- Garlic cloves (8 chopped)
- Butter (2 tablespoons)
- Cream (0.25 cup)
- Water (0.25 cup)

What to do:

1. Prepare the Marinade: Add all of the fixings using a whisk. Add the chicken and marinate for ½ hour at room temperature. (Place it in the refrigerator if it will take longer.)
2. Choose the saute button and add the butter to melt. Saute the garlic for 2-3 minutes.
3. Toss in the chicken. Reserve the marinade. Lightly brown the chicken. Pour in the water and marinade into the pot and secure the lid. Cook for 10 minutes and check the temperature. (Internal temperature must be 165° Fahrenheit/74° Celsius.)
4. Plate the chicken. Pour the cream into the Instant Pot, mixing well.
5. Serve with the sauce and enjoy.

Lemon Rotisserie Chicken

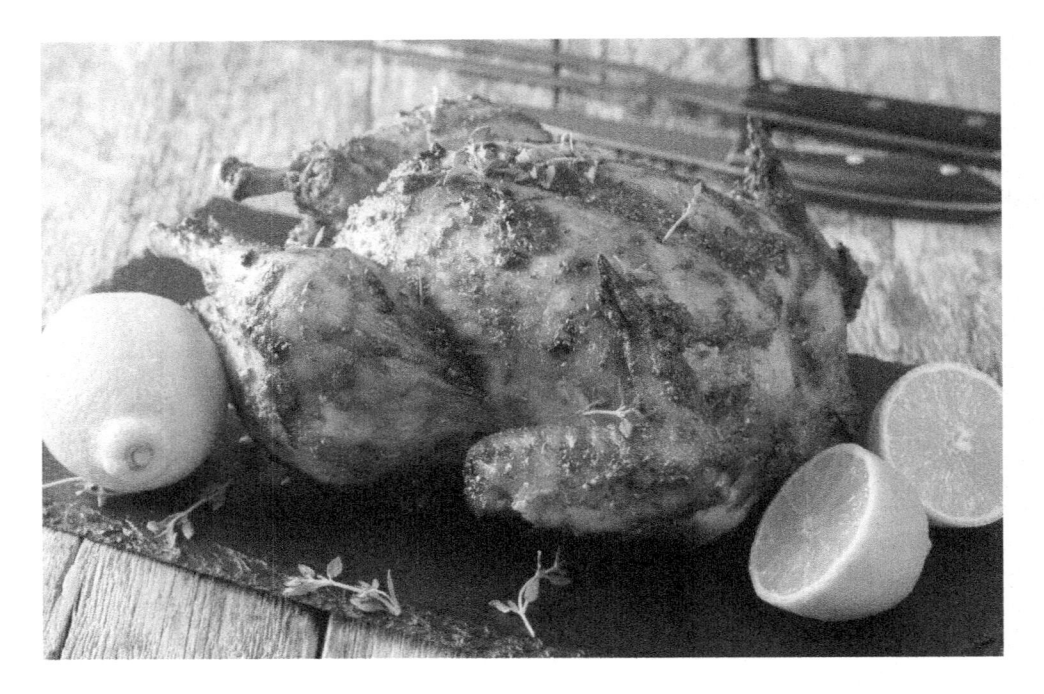

Yields: 6 Servings
Total prep & cooking time: 40 minutes
Nutrition Facts: Calories: 284 | Fat: 18.8 g | Protein: 25.7 g | Net Carbs: 2.9 g

What to use:

- Whole chicken (2.5 pounds)
- Olive oil (2 tablespoons)
- Paprika (1 teaspoon)
- Garlic powder (1 teaspoon)
- Chicken broth (1 cup)
- Salt (1.5 teaspoons)
- Black pepper (.5 teaspoon)
- Lemon (4 wedges)

What to do:

1. Thoroughly rinse the chicken - dab it using a paper towel till it's somewhat dry. Insert the lemon wedges into the cavity of the bird.
2. Choose the sauté mode in the Instant Pot.
3. Whisk the garlic powder with pepper, salt, oil, and paprika in a dish. Rub the top of the chicken (breast side down) using ½ of the spice mixture.
4. Sauté them for three to four minutes.
5. Rub the rest on the other half and flip, cooking one more minute.
6. Scoop the chicken into a container and arrange the trivet in the pot. Put the

chicken back (breast side down), and cover with the broth.
7. Secure the lid and set the timer for 20 minutes. Natural release the pressure at the end of the cooking cycle. Serve.

Whole Chicken & Gravy

Yields: 12 Servings
Total prep & cooking time: 45 minutes
Nutrition Facts: Calories: 450| Fat: 30.2 g | Protein: 34.5 g |Net Carbs: 0.7 g

What to use:

- Whole chicken (6.5 pounds)
- Olive oil (2 tablespoons)
- Onion powder (.5 teaspoon)
- Black pepper and salt (.5 teaspoon of each)
- Dried Italian seasonings (1 teaspoon)
- Garlic powder (.5 teaspoon)
- Chicken broth - low-sodium (1.5 cups)
- Guar gum (2 teaspoons)

What to do:

1. Rub oil (1 tbsp.) over the entire chicken and the rest of the oil into the Instant Pot. Combine the dry seasonings and sprinkle over the entire chicken.
2. Use the saute function to warm the oil, adding the chicken – breast side down. Let it sauté for five minutes, flip, and empty in the chicken broth.
3. Secure the top and set the timer for 40 minutes (manually). When done, simply quick-release the pressure.
4. Add the chicken to a bowl and prepare the gravy with guar gum in the hot broth. Stir until thickened. You can add another teaspoon if it isn't thick as you like it.
5. Serve with gravy and a sprinkle of chopped parsley.

Pork

Carnitas

Yields: 11 Servings
Total prep & cooking time: 1 hour 16 minutes
Nutritional Facts: Calories: 160 | Protein: 20 g | Fat: 7 g|Net Carbohydrates: 1 g

What to use:

- Shoulder blade roast – trimmed & boneless (2.5 pounds)
- Kosher salt (2 teaspoons)
- Black pepper (as desired)
- Cumin (1.5 teaspoons)
- Garlic (6 minced cloves)
- Sazon GOYA (.5 teaspoon)
- Dry oregano (0.25 teaspoon)
- Reduced-sodium chicken broth/homemade (0.75 cup)
- Bay leaves (2)
- Chipotle peppers in adobo sauce (2-3 or as desired)
- Dry adobo seasoning – ex. Goya (0.25 teaspoon)
- Garlic powder (.5 teaspoon)

What to do:

1. Prepare the roast with pepper and salt. Sear it for about five minutes in a skillet.
2. Let it cool and insert the garlic slivers into the roast using a blade (approximately one-inch deep). Season with garlic powder, Sazon, cumin, oregano, and adobo.
3. Arrange the chicken in the Instant Pot cooker. Pour in the broth, chipotle peppers, and bay leaves. Stir and secure the lid. Prepare using high pressure for 50 minutes (meat button).
4. Natural release the pressure and shred the pork. Combine with the juices and discard the bay leaves.
5. Add a bit more cumin and adobo if needed. Stir well and serve.

Chipotle Pork Roast

Yields: 4 Servings
Total prep & cooking time: 1 hour 22 minutes
Nutritional Facts: Calories: 460 | Protein: 40 g | Fat: 31 g|Net Carbs: 4 g

What to use:

- Diced tomatoes – canned okay (7.25 ounces)
- Bone broth (6 ounces)
- Mild diced canned green chilis (2 ounces)
- Pork roast (2 pounds)
- Onion powder (.5 teaspoon)
- Chipotle powder (1 teaspoon)
- Cumin (.5 teaspoon)

What to do:

1. Combine all of the ingredients in your Instant Pot.
2. Close the top of the pot and use the manual setting for 60 minutes.
3. Do a natural release of the pressure. Serve and enjoy.

Pork Ribs

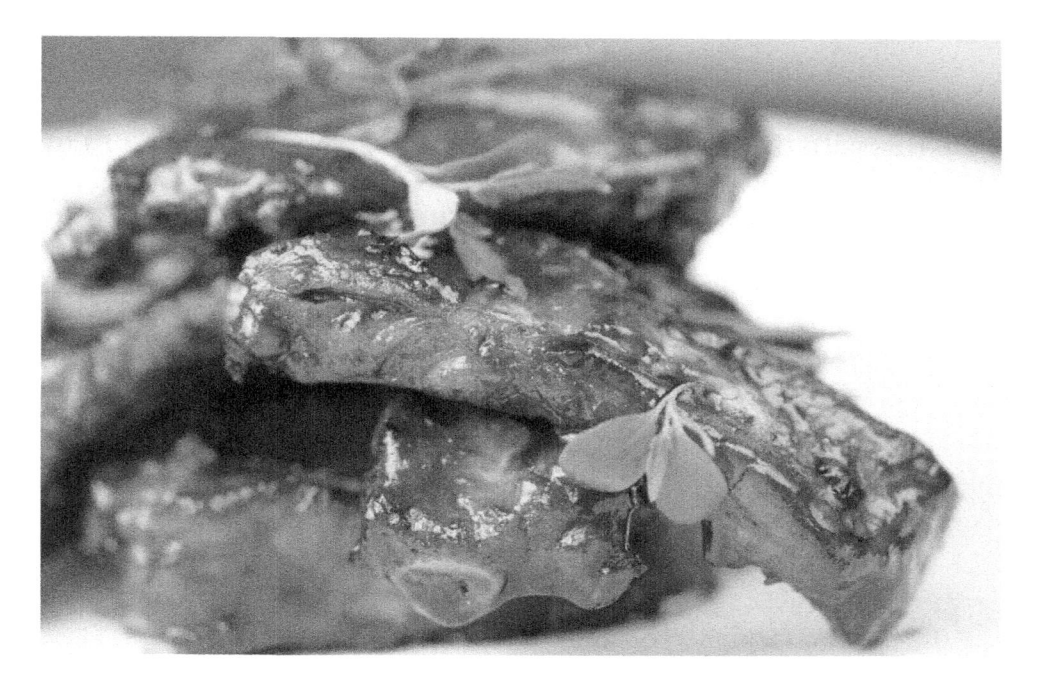

Yields: 6 Servings
Total preparation & cook time: 1 hr. 20 min.
Nutritional Facts: Calories: 387 | Proteins: 27 g | Fat: 29 g|Net Carbohydrates: 2 g

What to use:

- Country-style pork ribs (5-pound package)

What to use for the Rub:

- Erythritol/another sweetener (1 tablespoon)
- Spices: Paprika - Garlic powder - Onion powder (1 teaspoon each)
- Ground coriander (.5 teaspoon)
- Allspice (.5 teaspoon)
- Black pepper (.5 teaspoon)

What to use for the Sauce:

- Reduced-sugar/homemade (0.5 cup)
- Erythritol/your favorite sweetener (2 tablespoons)
- Water (0.5 cup)
- Red wine vinegar (2 tablespoons)
- Onion powder (0.5 teaspoon)
- Allspice (0.5 tablespoon)
- Liquid smoke (0.25 cup)

- Mustard (0.5 tablespoon)
- Optional: Xanthan gum (0.25 teaspoon)

What to do:

1. Rub the ribs with the combined seasonings and stack in the Instant Pot. Mix the sauce fixings and pour over the ribs.
2. Secure the lid and set it for 35 minutes (manually) under high pressure.
3. Natural-release the pressure and place the ribs in a container to keep warm.
4. Whisk in the xanthan gum (if using) and cook the juices for ten minutes using the saute function.
5. Serve and enjoy!

Pork Veggies & Noodles

Yields: 6 Servings
Total prep & cooking time: 20 minutes
Nutrition Facts: Calories: 241 | Protein: 15 g | Fat: 18 g|Net Carbohydrates: 3 g

What to use:

- Oil (1 tablespoon)
- Ground pork (1 pound)
- Chopped bell peppers (1 cup)
- Garlic (2 cloves)
- Onion (0.5 cup - chopped)
- Chopped baby spinach (4 cups)
- Shirataki noodles (2 packages)
- Grated parmesan cheese (.5 cup)

What to do:

1. Prepare the Instant Pot using the sauté mode.
2. Pour in the oil once it is heated.
3. Place the pork in the cooker and sauté it till it is slightly browned. Add the garlic, onions, peppers, and spinach. Scrape the browning bits from the bottom and secure the lid.
4. Use the high-pressure setting for three minutes and quick-release the pressure. Empty the sauce over the noodles and garnish with the cheese.

Spicy Pork – Korean Style

Yields: 4 Servings
Total prep & cooking time: 40 minutes
Nutrition Facts: Calories: 189| Fat: 10 g | Protein: 15 g |Net Carbs: 9g

What to use:

- Pork shoulder (1 pound)
- Onion (1 thinly sliced)
- Minced ginger and garlic (1 tablespoon of each)
- Rice wine (1 tablespoon)
- Soy sauce (1 tablespoon)
- Sesame oil (1 tablespoon)
- Splenda (2 packs)
- Cayenne (1 teaspoon)
- Gochugaru Chili flakes (2 tablespoons)
- Water (0.25 cups)

What to use for the Finishing:

- Sliced green onion (0.25 cup)
- Sesame seeds (1 tablespoon)
- Onion (1 thinly sliced)

What to do:

1. Cut the pork into ¼-½- inch slices and combine with its marinade fixings into a container. Wait for about 1 hour to 24 hours. When ready to cook, use the high-pressure setting for 20 minutes. Natural release.
2. Use a cast-iron skillet for cooking the thinly sliced onion and pork cubes. Once the pan is hot, just empty in the sauce, and mix with the pork.
3. When the sauce has cooled down, the onions will be soft. Toss the green onions and sesame seeds and serve.

Beef

Bacon Burger Cabbage Stir Fry

Yields: 10 serving
Total prep & cooking time: minutes
Nutrition Facts: Calories: 357 | Protein: 32 g | Net Carbs: 4.5 g | Fat: 22 g

What to use:

- Ground beef (1 pound)
- Bacon (1 pound)
- Small onion (1)
- Minced garlic (3 cloves)
- Cabbage (1 pound or 1 small head)
- Black pepper (.25 teaspoon)
- Sea salt (.5 teaspoon)

What to do:

1. Dice the bacon and onion.
2. Combine the bacon and beef in a wok or oversized skillet. Prepare until done and store in a bowl to keep warm.
3. Mince the onion and garlic. Toss both into the hot grease.
4. Slice and toss in the cabbage with pepper and salt - stir-fry until wilted.
5. Blend in the meat and combine. Serve as desired.

Beef Stroganoff

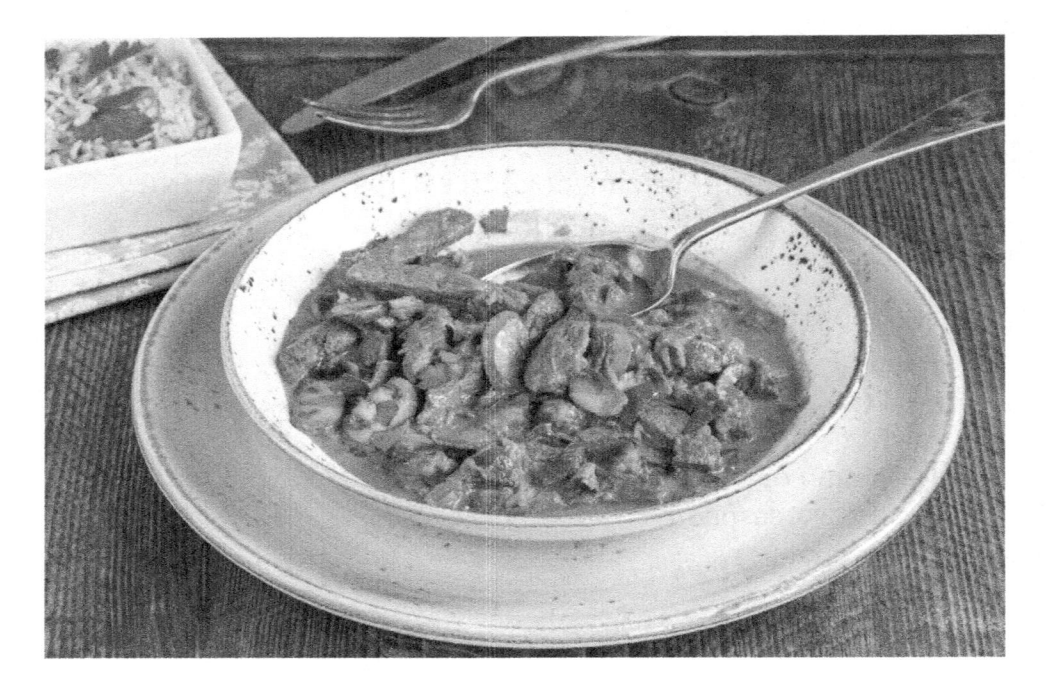

Yields: 1 serving
Total prep & cooking time: minutes
Nutrition Facts: Calories: 447 | Protein: 39 g | Net Carbs: 6 g | Fat: 28 g

What to use:

- Lean ground beef (1 pound)
- Sliced mushrooms (8 ounces)
- Minced cloves of garlic (2)
- Butter (2 tablespoons)
- Sour cream (1.25 cups)
- Water or dry white wine (.33 cup)
- Lemon juice (1 teaspoon)
- Dried parsley (1 teaspoon)
- Paprika (.25 teaspoon)
- *Optional:* Freshly chopped parsley (1 tablespoon)

What to do:

1. Warm a skillet to sauté the onions and garlic using one tablespoon of butter.
2. Mix the beef into the pan, and sprinkle with pepper and salt if desired. Cook until done and set to the side.
3. Add the remainder of the butter, mushrooms, and the wine/water to the pan.
4. Cook until half of the liquid is reduced and the mushrooms are soft.

5. Take them away from the heat and add the paprika and sour cream.
6. On low heat, stir in the meat and lemon juice. Use additional spices for flavoring if desired.

Greek Meatballs with Tomato Sauce

Yields: 6 Servings
Total prep & cooking time: 40 minutes
Nutrition Facts: Calories: 261| Fat: 16 g | Protein: 15 g |Net Carbs: 12 g

What to use for the Meatballs:

- Ground beef (1 pound)
- Egg (1 slightly beaten)
- Onion (.5 cup - finely chopped)
- Parsley (.25 cup - chopped)
- Arborio rice (.33 cup)
- Pepper and salt (as desired)

What to use for the Sauce:

- Water (1 cup)
- Diced tomatoes (14 ounces)
- Smoked paprika (.5 teaspoon)
- Dried oregano (1 teaspoon)
- Cinnamon (.5 teaspoon)
- Ground cloves (0.25 teaspoon)
- Pepper and salt (to your liking)

What to do:

1. Mix all of the meatballs fixings, shaping into eight to ten balls. Arrange in a single layer in the pot.
2. Mix the sauce components in a dish and pour over the prepared meatballs.
3. Program the Instant Pot for 15 minutes under high-pressure and release the pressure with the natural-release option.
4. Remove the meatballs and blend the sauce until smooth with an immersion blender.
5. Pour over the meatballs, garnish, and serve.

Italian Meatballs

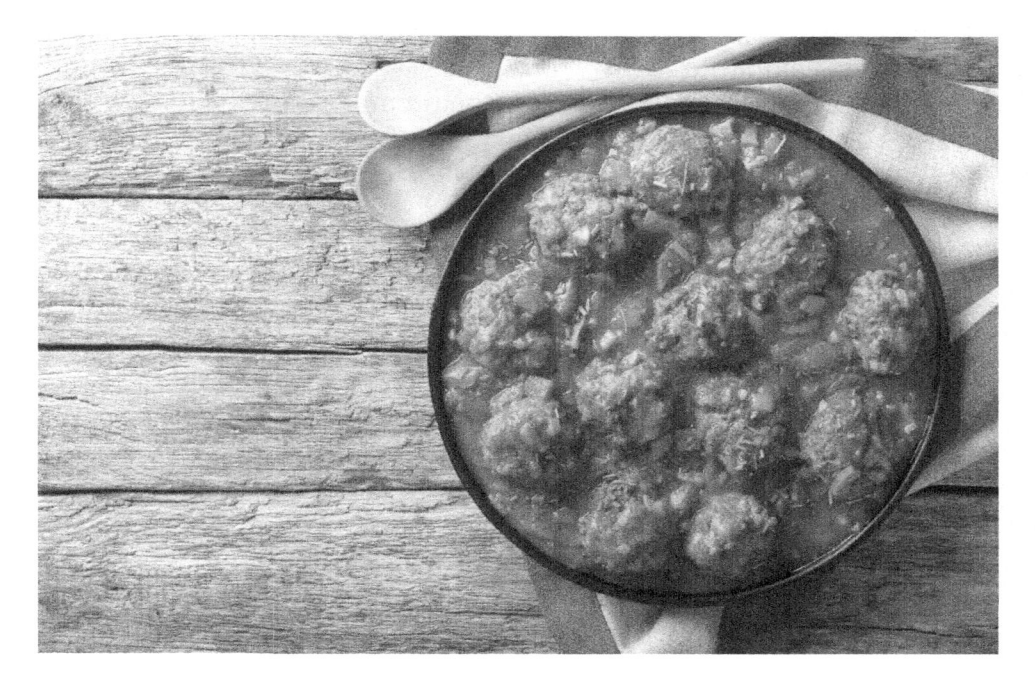

Yields: 5 Servings
Total prep & cooking time: 35 minutes
Nutrition Facts: Calories: 455| Fat: 33 g | Protein: 34 g |Net Carbs: 5 g

What to use for the Meatballs:

- Ground beef – lean (1.5 pounds)
- Freshly chopped parsley (2 tablespoons)
- Eggs (2)
- Almond flour (.5 cup)
- Grated parmesan cheese (.75 cup)
- Garlic powder (.25 teaspoon)
- Dried onion flakes (1 teaspoon)
- Dried oregano (.25 teaspoon)
- Kosher salt (1 teaspoon)
- Black pepper (.25 teaspoon)
- Warm water (.33 cup)

What to use:

- Olive oil (1 teaspoon)
- Keto-friendly marinara sauce/sugar-free sauce (3 cups)

What to do:

1. Mix all of the meatball fixings and shape into 15 (2-inch) balls.
2. Add the oil to the Instant Pot and program the saute function. Brown the meatballs by leaving a ½-inch space between each one in the pot. You can also brown them in a skillet first.
3. Pour in the marinara sauce and secure the lid on low-pressure for 10 minutes.
4. Natural-release the pressure and serve the tasty treat.

Shepherd's Pie

Yields: 12 Servings
Total prep & cooking time: 45 minutes
Nutrition Facts: Calories: 303| Fat: 21.2 g | Protein: 21.5 g |Net Carbs: 4.1 g

What to use:

- Water (1 cup)
- Butter (4 tablespoons)
- Cauliflower (1 head)
- Cream cheese (4 ounces)
- Mozzarella (1 cup)
- Egg (1)
- Pepper and salt (as desired)
- Garlic powder (1 tablespoon)
- Ground beef (2 pounds)
- Frozen peas and carrots (2 cups of each)
- Mushrooms (8 ounces - sliced)
- Beef broth (1 cup)

What to do:

1. Pour the water into the Instant Pot and arrange the cauliflower on top with the leaves and stems removed.
2. Close the lid and set for five minutes using high pressure.
3. Quick-release and toss the cauliflower into a blender. Scoop the cream cheese, butter, mozzarella, egg, pepper, and salt into the blender and mix till it's smooth.
4. Drain the water from the Instant Pot. Toss in the beef, carrots, peas, garlic powder, and broth with a bit more pepper and salt to your liking.
5. Blend in the cauliflower mixture and cook ten minutes on high (manual function).
6. Serve when it's ready.

Steak & Cheese Pot Roast

Yields: 8 Servings
Total preparation & cooking time: 1 hour 15 minutes
Nutritional Facts: Calories: 425 | Protein: 46.1 g| Fat: 25.7 g |Net Carbohydrates: 3.5 g

What to use:

- Oil (1 tablespoon)
- Large onions (2 thinly sliced)
- Sliced mushrooms (8 ounces)
- Montreal steak seasoning/another favorite Keto choice (1-2 tablespoons)
- Butter (1 tablespoon)
- Beef stock (.5 cup)
- Chuck roast (3 pounds)
- Optional: Keto cheese of choice 'add the carbs'

What to do:

1. Program the Instant Pot to saute and pour in the oil.
2. Rub the roast with the seasoning. Saute 1-2 minutes per side. Remove and add the butter and onions. Toss in the mushrooms, peppers, stock, and roast.
3. Choose the manual high-pressure for 35 minutes and natural release.
4. Shred the meat, sprinkle with cheese, and use as desired.

Other Favorites
Mutton Curry

Yields: 4 servings
Total prep & cooking time: 40 minutes
Nutrition Facts: Calories: 253| Fat: 13.5 g | Protein: 24.65g |Net Carbs: 6.34 g

What to use:

- Oil/ghee (3 tablespoons)
- Mutton bone-in (1 pound into 1-2-inch bits)
- Onion (1 large @ 11 ounces - finely chopped)
- Optional: Green chili (1)
- Garlic and ginger (.5 tablespoon of each - minced)
- Tomato (1 medium - chopped)
- Lemon juice (1 tablespoon)
- To Garnish: Cilantro

What to use: Spices:

- Salt (1 teaspoon)
- Coriander (2 teaspoons)
- Red chili powder - cayenne (1 teaspoon)
- Bay leaf (1)
- Garam masala (1 teaspoon)
- Black cardamom (2)
- Turmeric (0.25 teaspoon)
- Black peppercorns & cloves (6 of each)
- Cumin seeds (.5 teaspoon)
- Cinnamon stick (1 @ 1-inch)

What to do:

1. Use the saute function in the Instant Pot and pour in the oil. Fold in the whole spices and sauté them for ½ minute. Stir in the onions, green chilis, and garlic.
2. Sauté them for four minutes.
3. Blend in the spices and chopped tomatoes, stirring for another two minutes.
4. Stir in the mutton and mix well, sautéing for another two minutes.
5. Close the lid and change to the meat function for 20 minutes.
6. Natural-release the pressure and add the lemon juice. Garnish with the mutton curry and cilantro. Serve.

Chapter 8: Keto Sides & Snacks

Sides

Baked Zucchini Noodles With Feta

Yields: 3 servings
Total prep & cooking time: minutes
Nutrition Facts: Calories: 105 | Protein: 4 g | Net Carbs: 5 g | Fat: 8 g

What to use:

- Quartered plum tomato (1)
- Spiralized zucchini (2)
- Feta cheese (8 cubes)
- Pepper and salt (1 teaspoon each)
- Olive oil (1 tablespoon)

What to do:

1. Lightly grease a roasting pan with a spritz of oil.
2. Set the oven temperature to reach 375° Fahrenheit/191° Celsius.
3. Slice the noodles with a spiralizer and add to the prepared pan with olive oil and tomatoes. Sprinkle it with pepper and salt.
4. Bake for 10 to 15 minutes. Transfer from the oven and add the cheese cubes, tossing to combine. Serve.

Cauliflower Fried "Rice"

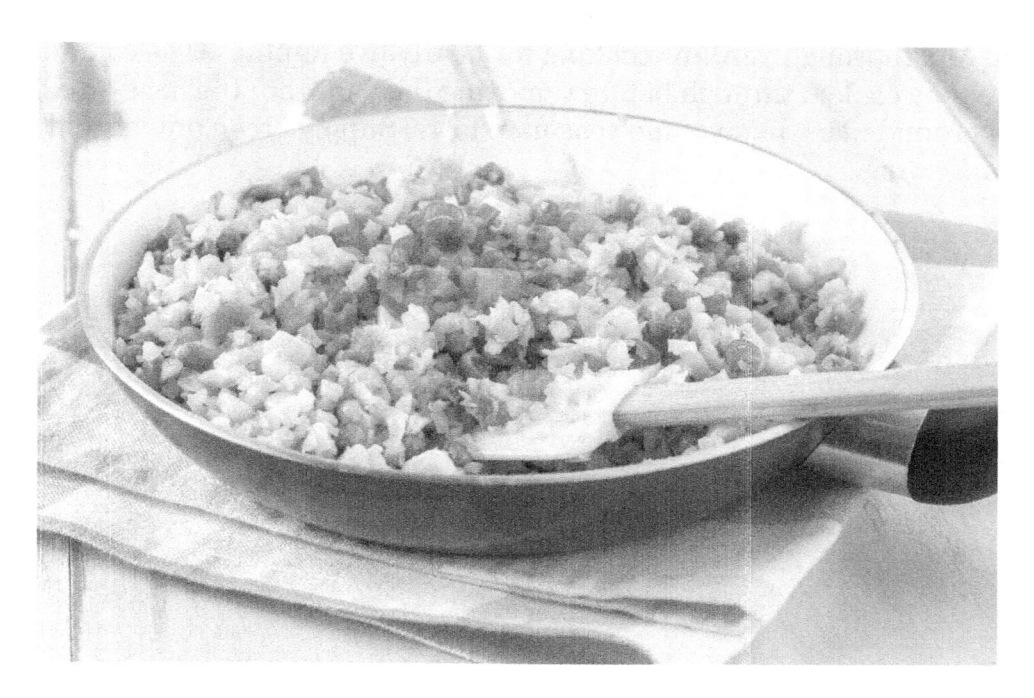

Yields: 4 servings
Total preparation & cooking time: ½ hour
Nutrition Facts: Calories: 152 | Protein: 6 g | Net Carbs: 18 g | Fat: 7 g

What to use:

- Cauliflower (1 head)
- Broccoli (1 head)
- Onion (diced) (1 medium-sized)
- Coconut oil (2 tablespoons)
- Carrot sticks (1 cup)
- Ginger (grated) (2 tablespoons)
- Water (2 to 3 tablespoons)
- Coconut aminos or Tamari (0.33 cup)
- Ground black pepper (a dash)
- Chopped cilantro (.5 cup)
- Thinly sliced green onions (0.25 cup)

What to do:

1. Warm a pan using the medium temperature setting on the stovetop. Pour in the oil to heat. Toss the onions into this pan and sauté them till they're softened.
2. To the pan with the heated coconut oil, add the water, carrot sticks, and broccoli. Add the water, broccoli, and carrot sticks. Place a lid over the pan and steam the vegetables until they become soft.

3. Push the veggies to one side of the skillet and add the riced cauliflower, ginger, and soy sauce. Let heat for a moment, and combine all of the ingredients in the pan. Mix thoroughly. Allow cooking for nearly five minutes. The cauliflower should be cooked through before removing the pan from the heat.
4. Add ground black pepper and season to taste. Supply green onions and cilantro upon serving.

Crispy Cauliflower Zucchini Fritters

Yields: 8 cakes
Total prep & cooking time: 10 minutes
Nutrition Facts: Calories: 54| Protein: 4 g | Fat: 2 g| Net Carbohydrates: 2 g

What to use:

- Your preferred flour (almond, coconut, etc.) (.25 cup)
- Zucchini (2 whole medium-sized)
- Cauliflower (chopped – or use frozen steamable broccoli) (.5 head, or about 3 cups)
- Black pepper (.25 teaspoon)
- Salt (.5 teaspoon)
- Coconut oil (1 tablespoon)

What to do:

1. Allow the cauliflower to steam for close to five minutes. The cauliflower should become tender but not soft and mushy.
2. Making use of a food processor, grate the zucchini directly into the bowl of the processor.
3. Add the steamed cauliflower to the zucchini in the bowl. Pulse the food processor until the zucchini and cauliflower resemble small chunks. Do not process this for too long, or the mixture will become mushy.
4. Wring as much moisture out of the vegetables as you can using a towel. Be sure to do this over the sink. Place the vegetables into a bowl, into which you will add the salt, flour, pepper, and any other seasonings. Stir all of these together until they are all combined. Once the ingredients have been mixed thoroughly, form the resulting mixture into small patties.
5. Warm a big skillet using a medium-temperature setting and heat the coconut oil. Arrange the cakes in the oil to cook for nearly three minutes.
6. Flip over the patties and then cook for another three minutes. Serve the cakes piping hot.

Pad Thai with Zucchini Noodles

This dinner is light but still filling. It's full of herbs, crunchy peanuts, and fresh vegetables - including zucchini noodles in place of carb-filled noodles.

Yields: 2 generous servings
Total prep & cooking time: 10 minutes
Nutrition Facts: Calories: 290 | Protein: 17 g | Net Carbs: 4 g | Fat: 10 g

What to use:

- Zucchini (3 whole, spiralized, or you can buy zucchini noodles at the store)
- Peanut oil (2 tablespoons)
- Bell pepper (1 whole)
- Garlic cloves (3 whole)
- Small onion (1 whole, thinly sliced)
- Ginger (1 tablespoon)
- Carrots (2 whole)
- Soy sauce (2 tablespoons)
- Rice vinegar (1 tablespoon)
- Fish sauce (2 tablespoons)
- Basil leaves (0.25 cup, chopped)
- Chili flakes (1 teaspoon)
- Cilantro leaves (0.5 cup - chopped)
- Brown sugar (1 tablespoon)
- Lime (0.5 of a whole, juiced)
- Scallions (3 whole, sliced thinly)
- Roasted peanuts (0.3 cup - chopped)

What to do:

1. Microwave the zucchini noodles in a glass bowl for about 20 seconds until they are warm and slightly softened. Put them into a strainer and allow the liquid to drain out of them.
2. Warm the oil in a big frying pan on the stovetop burner using a med-high temperature setting. Slice and add the onion and sauté it till it's softened and slightly translucent (3 min.).
3. Thinly slice and add the bell pepper. Mince and add the garlic and ginger, cooking for an additional two minutes and stirring throughout this time.
4. Shave the carrots with a vegetable peeler and add them to the pan, stirring to combine.
5. Whisk the soy sauce with rice vinegar, sugar, fish sauce, lime juice, and chili flakes till they're mixed and thoroughly combined. Fold in the zucchini noodles and sauce to the pan - tossing to cover.
6. Gently fold in the cilantro, scallions, basil, and peanuts. Serve immediately.

Roasted Cabbage With Lemon

This recipe makes an excellent side dish for a variety of meals. It's flavorful, salty, and lemony and tastes fresh and delicious.

Yields: 4 servings
Total prep & cooking time: 35 minutes
Nutrition Facts: Calories: 78 | Protein: 1 g | Net Carbs: 2 g | Fat: 7 g

What to use:

- Cabbage (1 large head)
- Lemon juice (fresh, 2-3 tablespoons)
- Olive oil (2 tablespoons)
- Black pepper and salt (a pinch, or as desired)

What to do:

1. Allow ample time for your oven to preheat to 450° Fahrenheit/232° Celsius.
2. Cut the cabbage into eight wedges and arrange in a roasting pan sprayed with a tiny bit of olive oil.
3. Thoroughly whisk the oil and lemon juice in a mixing container. Use a pastry brush to brush the cabbage wedges with the oil-lemon juice mixture. Sprinkle them using a bit of pepper and salt. Flip the wedges and repeat this process.
4. Put the roasting pan into the preheated oven.
5. Set a timer to roast the cabbage (15 min.).
6. Turn the wedges carefully, put the cabbage pan back into the oven, and roast the cabbage for another 15 minutes.
7. Serve while hot.

Spaghetti Squash with Tomato & Mushroom

Yields: 4 servings
Total prep & cooking time: 40 minutes
Nutrition Facts: Calories: 173 | Protein: 4 g | Net Carbs: 6 g | Fat: 12 g

Like regular spaghetti, but much healthier, spaghetti squash will take the place of carb-filled spaghetti and still fills that craving for noodles. Spaghetti squash seems intimidating initially, but it's easy to cook and is delicious. It even keeps nicely in the fridge and tastes great the next day!

You can cook the spaghetti squash in a couple of ways:

You can cook it in an oven preheated to 400° Fahrenheit/204° Celsius if you have time. Cut the squash from the stem to the base and use a spoon to remove the seeds. Coat the inside of the squash in olive oil (about one tablespoon per side). You can add herbs as well. Place the squash on a baking tray lined with parchment paper (cut-side facing downward).

Bake for about an hour until the cut side of the squash is beginning to turn golden. Remove the "spaghetti" with a fork.

If you're short on time, you can cook spaghetti squash in the microwave. Pierce the squash with a sharp knife several times. Microwave it whole for a few minutes - this will make it easier to cut. Cut the squash from the stem to the base and scoop out the seeds. Put the squash cut-side down in a glass pie plate with a little water and microwave for a few minutes at a time, until it's soft and the "spaghetti" can be easily removed using a fork.

What to use:

- Spaghetti squash (2 whole, about 6 cups once prepared)
- Tomatoes (2 cups - diced)
- Garlic (4 cloves -minced)
- Onions (0.3 cup -chopped)
- Pine nuts - toasted is best (0.25 cup)
- Mushrooms (sliced) (8 ounces)
- Olive oil (3 tablespoons)
- Red pepper flakes (optional) (a pinch)
- Fresh basil (1 handful - chopped)
- Black pepper and salt (season as desired)

What to do:

1. Prepare the spaghetti squash according to your preferred method, remove the "spaghetti" portion of the squash, and set it to the side for later.

2. In a pan over a stove burner set to medium heat, place the oil and allow it to become warm. Put the mushrooms and onions into the oiled pan and constantly stir them until they begin to soften slightly. (This should take nearly four minutes.)
3. Toss in the minced garlic and sauté it while stirring for about another two minutes. Place the tomatoes into this pan and cook for a while longer, also while stirring.
4. The spaghetti squash will be placed into the pan and all of the ingredients tossed until they are combined. Heat until the squash becomes hot and the vegetables are distributed evenly throughout the mixture.
5. Transfer the pan to the countertop. Top the mixture with the chopped basil, salt, pepper, a pinch of pepper flakes, and pine nuts. Serve and enjoy.

Tofu Fries - Keto-Friendly

You will simply love these tofu fries packed with protein and full of flavor with a crunchy outside and delicious center. You'll probably like these even if you don't like tofu, so definitely give them a try.

Yields: 4 servings
Total prep & cooking time: 70 minutes
Nutritional Facts: Calories: 132 | Protein: 7 g | Net Carbs: 3 g | Fat: 10 g

What to use:

- Tofu - extra-firm (1 package, drained & pressed)
- Olive oil (2 tablespoons)
- Oregano (.5 teaspoon)
- Basil (.5 teaspoon)
- Garlic powder (.25 teaspoon)
- Paprika (.25 teaspoon)
- Onion powder (.25 teaspoon)
- Black pepper & salt (a pinch, or to taste)
- Cayenne pepper (.25 teaspoon)

What to do:

1. Warm the oven to 375° Fahrenheit/191° Celsius.
2. Cover a baking tray using a sheet of parchment baking paper and set it aside.
3. Combine the oil, spices, and herbs in a mixing container.
4. Slice your drained and pressed tofu into long strips, about ¼ of an inch thick.
5. Cover the tofu strips in the olive oil mixture, and arrange them on the prepared baking tray.
6. Bake in a preheated oven (20 min.).
7. Flip the tofu fries and bake till done (20 min.) to serve.

Snacks

Baked Zucchini Chips

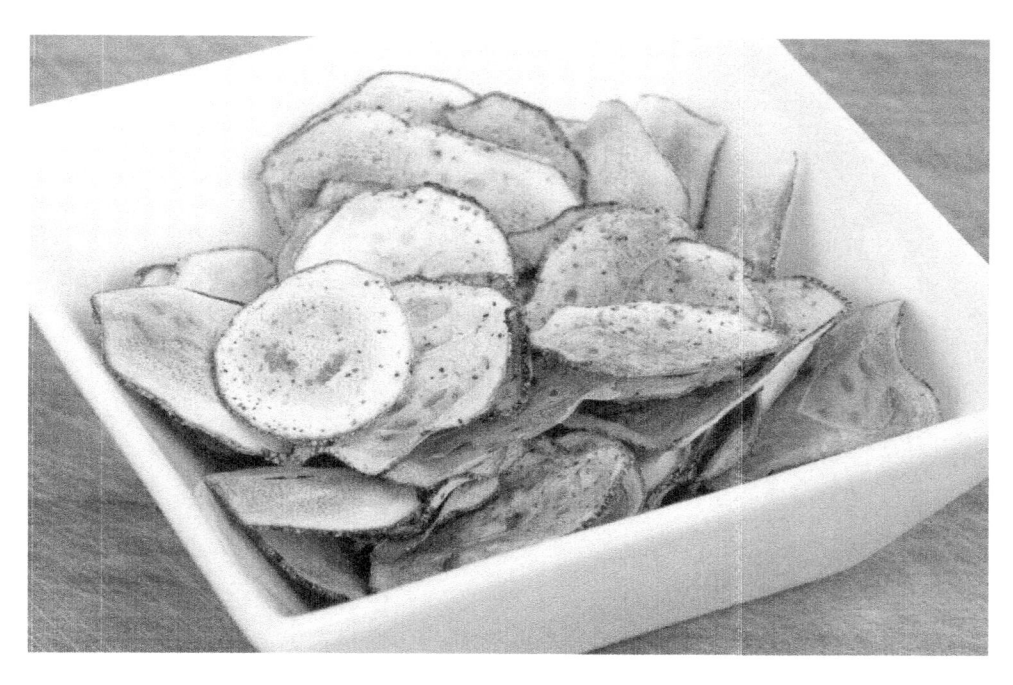

These healthy, crispy chips will satisfy your craving for a crunchy snack without all the potato chips' starch. The trick to making these crisp up in the oven is to slice your zucchini as thinly as possible. A mandolin slicer will be very helpful for this but isn't 'absolutely' necessary.

Yields: 8 servings
Total prep & cooking time: 2 hours and 10 minutes (largely unattended)
Nutrition Facts: Calories: 23 | Protein: 1 g | Net Carbs: 1 g | Fat: 2 g

What to use:

- Zucchini (2 whole medium-sized)
- Oil (olive or avocado) (1 tablespoon)
- Salt (.5 teaspoon)

What to do:

1. Warm the oven to 200° Fahrenheit/93° Celsius.
2. Slice your zucchini as thin as you can (preferably about ⅛ inch thickness).
3. Toss the zucchini in the oil until it's evenly coated. Sprinkle on the salt.
4. If you have cookie baking racks, use those. If not, use a baking tray (they won't crisp up quite the same on a baking tray, but they'll still taste great!).

5. Bake the chips for 2 ½ hours, rotating the pans about halfway through. The chips are done when they're just beginning to crisp up. Open the oven door and let them cool this way. Serve and enjoy!

Cauliflower Hummus with Garlic

This hummus uses delicious roasted cauliflower instead of non-keto chickpeas, and it's wonderful. You only need a few ingredients and less than an hour to make it, and you'll be so glad you did.

Yields: 4 to 6 servings
Total prep & cooking time: 35 minutes
Nutrition Facts: Calories: 156 | Protein: 2.8 g | Fat: 14.7 g| Net Carbohydrates: 5.4 g

What to use:

- Cauliflower (1 head, large)
- Cloves of garlic (4 to 6 cloves as per your preference)
- Tahini (0.25 cup)
- Avocado oil (0.25 cup)
- Paprika (.5 teaspoon)
- Black pepper & salt (as desired)

What to do:

1. Preheat your oven to 425° Fahrenheit/218° Celsius - allow plenty of time for it to reach this temperature. Prepare the cauliflower.
2. Roast the cauliflower and cloves of garlic in the preheated oven (20 min.). Flip the vegetables and roast for another 15 to 20 minutes.
3. Transfer the pan to the countertop to cool.
4. Toss each of the fixings into a food processor. Blend till they're incorporated and velvety smooth. You can alter the flavors to your liking with more lemon juice, salt, or pepper.

Delicious Guacamole

This guacamole is simple, delicious, and destined to be the best guacamole you've ever had. It only contains a few ingredients and is ready to eat in minutes. If you need to store it, place it in a container and pat it down firmly so that it's flat on top. Add a little water (about half an inch), put the lid on, and place it in the fridge. Enjoy it for about two to three days.

Yields: 4 servings
Total prep & cooking time: 10 minutes
Nutrition Facts: Calories: 184.8 | Protein: 2.5 g | Fat: 15.8 g | Net Carbohydrates: 12.3 g

What to use:

- Avocados (3 whole)
- Tomatoes (2 whole, we used Roma)
- Onion (0.5 of a whole small)
- Jalapeno pepper (1 whole, chopped, seeds removed)
- Cilantro (3 tablespoons, chopped)
- Garlic (2 cloves)
- Juice of 1 lime
- Salt (.5 teaspoon)

What to do:

1. Prepare the avocado. Put the avocado meat in a bowl and use a fork to mash it until it's as smooth or as chunky as you like.
2. Combine all of the fixings until they're thoroughly mixed.
3. That's it! Serve and enjoy!

Keto Seed Crackers

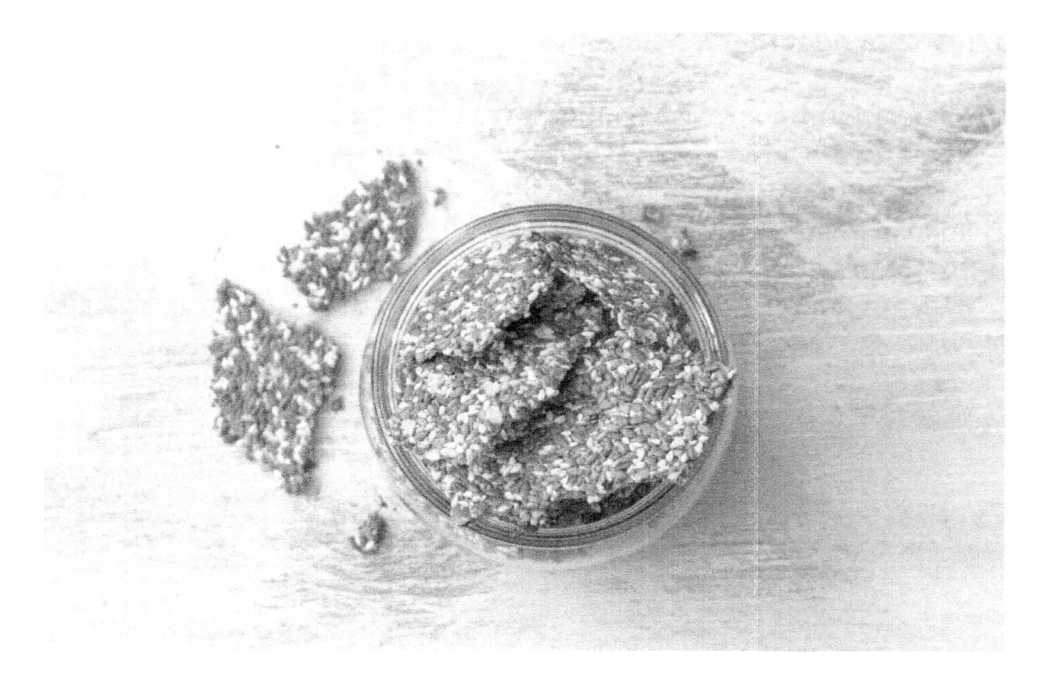

These simple crackers taste like a lot of work (but they're not!). The 3 hour cook time is mostly unattended – you just have to flip the mixture once, halfway through.

Yields: 10 servings
Total prep & cooking time: 3 hours and 3 minutes (largely unattended)
Nutrition Facts: Calories: 128 | Protein: 5.3 g | Fat: 9.4 g| Net Carbohydrates: 7.7 g

What to use:

- Whole flaxseeds (1 cup)
- Water (1 cup)
- Sunflower seeds (3 tablespoons)
- Hemp hearts (3 tablespoons)
- Salt (.5 teaspoon)
- Chia seeds (3 tablespoons)
- Your preferred blend of herbs and spices (ex. - dried rosemary, finely chopped) (3 tablespoons)
- Sesame seeds (3 tablespoons)

What to do:

1. Preheat your oven to 200° Fahrenheit/93° Celsius. Give it ample time to become this temperature.
2. Cover your baking tray using a layer of parchment baking paper to cover the entire surface and set aside.

3. Mix the flaxseeds and chia seeds in a bowl with the water. Mix well. Let the mixture sit for about 20 minutes.
4. Add the remainder of the fixings into the bowl and stir. Be sure it's mixed very well.
5. Spread the mixture onto the baking tray. Try to get it in as thin a layer as you can.
6. Bake them for 1½ hours - take the tray out of the oven. Using a spatula, flip the cracker sheet. It should still be fairly flexible and hold together during the flip. You can also place a new layer of parchment baking paper on top of the cracker, then flip the tray.
7. Bake for another 1½ hours - transfer the tray to the countertop and allow the crackers to cool completely on the tray. Break the cracker sheet into individual crackers and store them in a sealed container. They should stay good for about five to seven days.

Lettuce Wraps with Hemp Seed & Ginger

Yields: 4 servings
Total prep & cooking time: 10 minutes
Nutrition Facts: Calories: 382 | Protein: 14 g | Net Carbs: 13 g | Fat: 31 g

What to use for the sauce:

- Minced ginger (1 tablespoon)
- Keto maple syrup (1 tablespoon)
- Sesame oil (1 teaspoon)
- Brown rice vinegar (2 tablespoons)
- Tamari/coconut aminos (2 tablespoons)

For the filling:

- Chopped walnuts (1 cup)
- Hemp seeds (.5 cup)
- Chopped cucumber (.5 cup)
- Chopped carrots (0.25 cup)
- Dates (chopped) (2 whole)
- Lettuce leaves (a few)
- (Optional) Sesame seeds

What to do:

1. Into a bowl, stir all of the ingredients for the sauce together until combined well and set to the side.
2. Use different bowls to mix the chopped walnuts, hemp seeds, chopped carrots, chopped cucumber, and chopped dates. Once these are mixed, add the sauce mixture from the other bowl and stir the filling mixture together with the sauce until each piece is coated. Place the whole mixture into the fridge for at least an hour.
3. When the mixture has chilled, place spoonfuls of the filling onto the lettuce leaves. Sprinkle the sesame seeds over the top of the filling in the lettuce tacos, fold the lettuce leaves around the filling, and eat.

Low-Carb Almond Flour Crackers

If you miss having regular wheat crackers, you'll love these. These almond-flour crackers get as close to wheat crackers as possible on keto - and they taste great! They're surprisingly simple to prepare and only contain a handful of ingredients.

Yields: 6 servings
Total prep & cooking time: 25 minutes
Nutrition Facts: Calories: 151 | Protein: 4 g | Net Carbs: 6 g | Fat: 13 g

What to use:

- Sunflower seeds (2 tablespoons)
- Almond flour (1 cup)
- Water (2 tablespoons)
- Flax meal (1 tablespoon)
- Coconut oil (1 tablespoon)
- Salt (.75 tablespoon)

What to do:

1. Allow ample time for your oven to preheat to 350° Fahrenheit/177° Celsius.
2. Toss the dry fixings into a blender - mix till they're finely chopped. Mix in the water and coconut oil - pulse until the mixture forms a dough.
3. Press the mixture flat on a parchment paper sheet, then cover with another sheet of parchment and roll out dough. You want it to be about ⅛ inch thick (or even thinner if you can).
4. Cut into 1" squares (or desired shape) and sprinkle the salt on top.
5. Transfer chips to a baking tray and bake until the edges are crispy and brown (about 10-15 minutes). Let them cool on a rack and then separate. These keep best in the fridge but can be stored at room temperature for a couple of days.

Slow-Cooker Granola

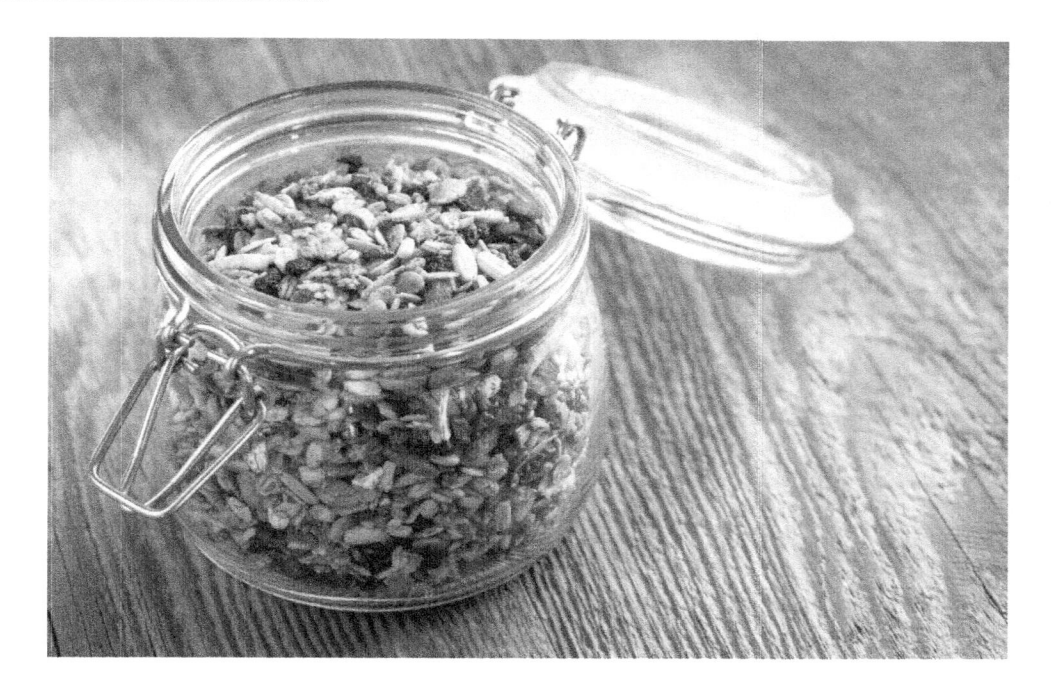

Yields: 14 servings
Total prep & cooking time: 3 hours and 5 minutes (largely unattended)
Nutrition Facts: Calories: 214 | Protein: 6 g | Net Carbs: 8 g | Fat: 18 g

What to use:

- Sunflower seeds (1 cup)
- Pumpkin seeds (.5 cup)
- Unsweetened, shredded coconut (.5 cup)
- Mixed nuts, preferably raw cashews, almonds, and walnuts, but any nuts you have on hand will work (2 cups)
- Sesame seeds (2 tablespoons)
- Dried orange zest (.5 teaspoon)
- Ground nutmeg and cardamom (0.25 teaspoon)
- Sugar-free maple syrup (2 teaspoons)
- Olive or coconut oil (2 teaspoons)

What to do:

1. Combine the sunflower seeds, pumpkin seeds, shredded coconut, mixed nuts, sesame seeds, dried orange zest, ground nutmeg, and cardamom into the same bowl and mix well.

2. Use a different bowl to mix the oil with the maple syrup. Combine this mixture into the container with the dry ingredients and mix to coat the dry ingredients well.
3. Add the mixture into your slow cooker. Set the time of your slow cooker for 3 hours. Check the time and stir the mixture every 45 minutes.
4. When the granola becomes crispy and golden, it will be ready.
5. Pour the granola from your slow cooker onto a cookie sheet and give it ample time to cool completely.
6. Store the granola in a tightly closed container to enjoy for up to two weeks.

Tasty Keto Vegan Granola

Yields: 5 servings
Total prep & cooking time: 20 minutes
Nutrition Facts: Calories: 196 | Protein: 6 g | Fat: 18 g | Net Carbohydrates: 6 g

What to use:

- Chopped mixed nuts (.5 cup)
- Almonds (1 cup)
- Blanched almond flour (.5 cup)
- Keto maple syrup (.33 cup)
- Unsweetened coconut - shredded (1 cup)

What to do:

1. Program the oven setting to 350° Fahrenheit/177° Celsius and carefully line a cookie sheet or baking tray with parchment baking paper - put it to the side
2. Toss all of the dry fixings in a big mixing container - mixing till incorporated. Drizzle the mixture with the keto maple syrup. Stir well to coat all dry ingredients with the syrup.
3. Retrieve your parchment-lined tray and spread the mixture out into one thin, even layer.
4. Put the baking tray in the oven to cook for ten minutes. Stir the mixture around with a spoon and then bake for another 15 minutes. The granola should begin to become golden brown.
5. The granola will need to cool completely. Afterward, break it up into chunks and then store it in a sealable airtight container. This granola can keep for no more than a month if it is stored appropriately.

Trail Mix with Coconut

This trail mix is a very healthy and extremely tasty little snack! It's a great blend of nuts, coconut, and cinnamon.

Yields: 26 servings (0.25 cup serving size)
Total prep & cooking time: 23 minutes
Nutrition Facts: Calories: 290| Protein:3 g | Net Carbs: 2 g | Fat: 22 g

What to use:

- Raw nuts - cashews - almonds & pecans (2 cups of each)
- Coconut shreds (1 cup)
- Cinnamon (1 tablespoon)
- Coconut oil (2 tablespoons, melted)
- Salt (2 teaspoons, or to taste)

What to do:

1. Allow plenty of time for your oven to become preheated to 350 F.
2. Put all ingredients into a mixing container and toss to combine.
3. Spread mix over a large baking sheet. Be sure to get it in one even layer.
4. In the oven that has been preheated, bake the tray for about 10 minutes, toss, and bake for another 10 minutes.
5. Let the trail mix cool completely before serving or storing.

Chapter 9: Keto Desserts

Chocolate Avocado Ice Cream

Missing ice cream? This treat is a great stand-in! It's rich and creamy, full of delicious flavors, and, best of all, it's healthy! It requires a bit of time and a little muscle, but it's a fun process that results in a fantastic dessert.

Yields: 3 cups
Total prep & cooking time: 2 hours and 15 minutes
Nutrition Facts: Calories: 278 | Protein: 3.06 g | Net Carbs: 12.19 g | Fat: 25.74 g

What to use:

- Full-fat coconut milk (1 15 ounce can)
- Vanilla extract (1 teaspoon)
- Your preferred granulated sweetener (.33 cup)
- Espresso powder (this is optional but makes it taste more chocolatey) (1 teaspoon)
- Sugar-free dark chocolate (3 ounces)
- Avocados (2 whole medium-sized)
- Ground cinnamon (1.5 teaspoons)
- Chipotle powder or chili powder for milder spice) (0.25 teaspoon)

What to do:

1. Whisk the coconut milk, sweetener, and espresso powder in a saucepan over a stove burner heated to medium heat. Simmer.
2. Transfer the pan from the heated stove - add the chocolate. Let it sit until the chocolate is melted. Whisk until smooth, adding in the vanilla extract along the way.
3. Put the avocados, chocolate mixture, chipotle, and cinnamon into a blender and puree till it's smooth. Pop it into the fridge to cool.
4. Transfer the mixture to a stainless steel baking dish and put it in the freezer. Check it after 45 minutes. It should be freezing around the edges. Take it out of the freezer, stir it vigorously with a spatula or beat with a handheld mixer, then return it to the freezer.
5. Check on the mixture every half hour, stirring each time vigorously. After about two to three hours, the ice cream should be set and ready to eat.

Chocolate Avocado Pudding

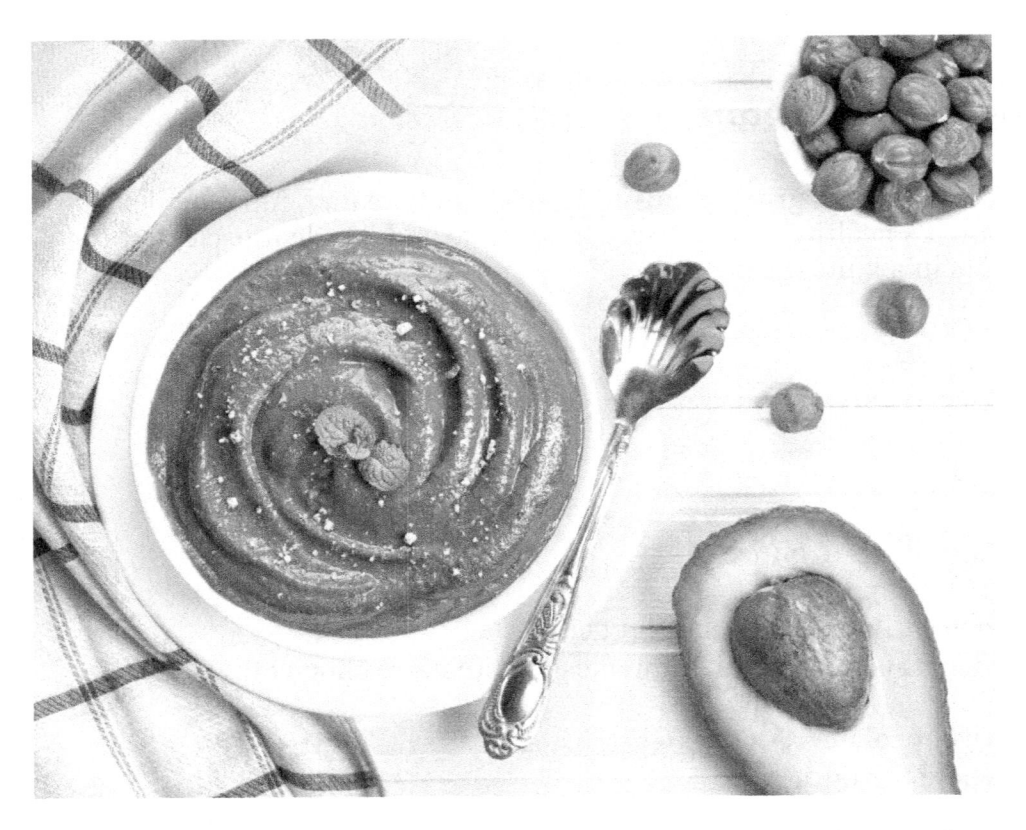

This pudding is so rich and creamy - also sugar-free. It's keto and vegan-friendly, and excellent for those on a gluten-free, dairy-free, paleo, or Atkins diet!

Yields: 3 servings
Total prep & cooking time: 5 minutes
Nutrition Facts: Calories: 288 | Protein: 5 g | Net Carbs: 12 g | Fat: 25 g

What to use:

- Almond milk (1.5 cups)
- Coconut cream (0.5 cup)
- Avocado (1 whole medium-sized)
- Cocoa powder - unsweetened (3 tablespoons)
- Stevia (or your preferred sweetener) (3 tablespoons)
- Almond and vanilla extracts (1 teaspoon of each)
- Unsweetened coconut flakes and sliced almonds for garnish (optional)

What to do:

1. Toss each of the fixings into your food processor - pulse till they become a smooth mixture.

2. Pour this mixture into serving bowls or little cups and cover with plastic wrap. Refrigerate until set for at least five hours. You can also let them sit overnight.
3. Top with coconut flakes and sliced almonds right before serving.

Chocolate Fat Bombs

These super-simple two-ingredient fat bombs are delicious!

Yields: about 24 servings
Total prep & cooking time: 5 minutes
Nutrition Facts: Calories: 132 | Protein: 4 g | Net Carbs: 5 g | Fat: 12 g

What to use:

- Almond butter/your favorite (1 cup)
- Keto-friendly chocolate chips (2 cups)

What to do:

1. Cover a plate or baking tray with parchment paper, being sure to cover the surface completely and thoroughly.
2. Combine your preferred nut butter with the chocolate chips in a bowl and microwave in 30-second increments. Stir after each increment and continue stirring and heating until the chocolate is melted and the ingredients are well-combined.
3. Whisk one last time and let cool. Use a cookie scoop or spoon to scoop 24-even scoops. Roll into balls and set on the parchment-lined tray. Place the tray in the freezer.
4. If you want, you can decorate with a simple drizzle. Melt some chocolate chips and use a fork to drizzle the melted chocolate over the fat bomb. You can also dunk the fat bomb into the melted chocolate for a completely coated chocolate bomb. Refrigerate until the chocolate firms up.

Crunchy Protein Bars

This filing is a healthy and protein-packed bar that's crunchy and crispy and sure to be a hit. Even better is that it only takes a few minutes to prepare!

Yields: 20 bars
Total prep & cooking time: 10 minutes
Nutritional Facts: Calories: 137 | Protein: 9 g | Fat: 10 g| Net Carbohydrates: 5 g

What to use:

- Coconut flour (0.75 cup)
- Chocolate chips (2 cups)
- Your preferred sticky sweetener (.5 cup)
- Smooth nut butter (2 cups)
- Roasted nuts or seeds (.5 cup)
- Your preferred protein powder (2 scoops)

What to do:

1. Cover an eight-inch pan using a sheet of parchment baking paper to completely cover and set to the side for later.
2. Combine your nut butter with syrup and mix until well combined. If you need to, you can heat the mixture for a few seconds in the microwave to make it easier to combine.
3. Add the dry ingredients and mix well, being sure all ingredients are combined.
4. Place the mixture in the lined pan and press firmly into place. Put the pan in the fridge until the mixture is firm.
5. Using a sharp knife, cut into 20 bars.
6. Melt the chocolate chips. Use two forks to dip each bar in the melted chocolate, being sure to coat evenly. Repeat until all the bars are covered and refrigerate them until the chocolate is firm.

Energy Balls

This super easy no-bake recipe needs just three ingredients to make delicious and filling energy balls. You can mess with the recipe a little by adding cocoa powder, nut butter, or a scoop of protein powder.

Yields: 40 energy balls
Total prep & cooking time: 10 minutes
Nutrition Facts: Calories: 57 | Protein: 2 g | Net Carbs: 3 g | Fat: 4 g

What to use:

- Smooth tahini (2 cups)
- Coconut flour (0.75 cup)
- Your preferred sticky syrup (.5 cup)

What to do:

1. Place your tahini in a big mixing container. If it's not smooth and easy to work with, microwave it for a few seconds to soften it up a bit.
2. Add the syrup and mix well.
3. Mix in the flour till each of the ingredients is combined. If the mixture is too thin, add more coconut flour.
4. Roll evenly-sized balls of the mixture between your palms and put them on a parchment-lined baking tray. Refrigerate till the balls are firm.

Key Lime Bars

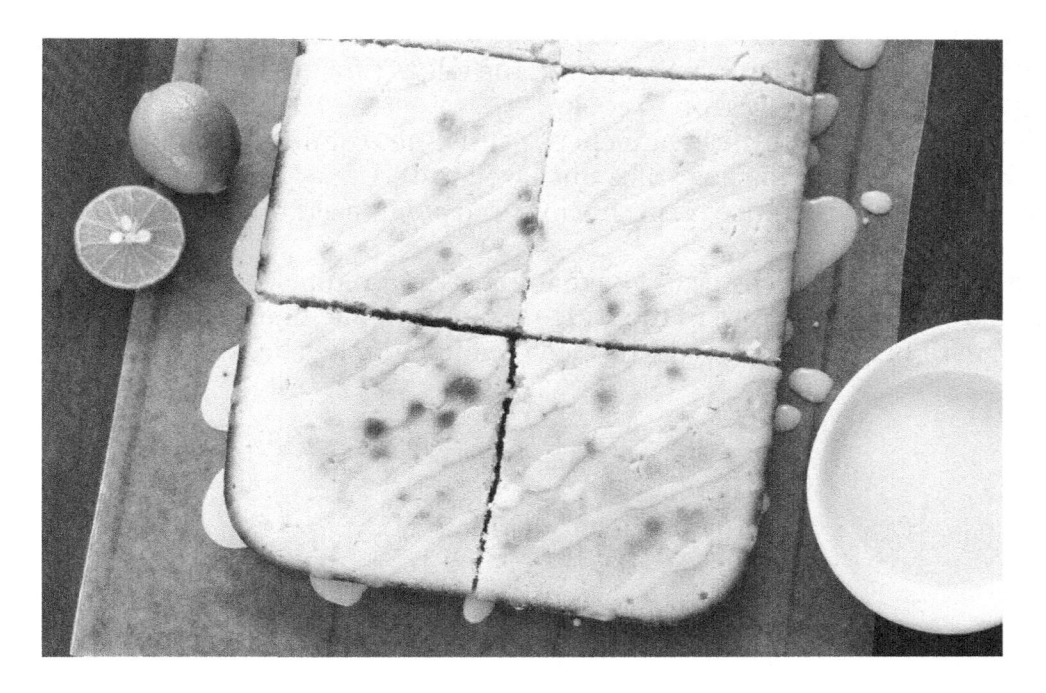

Yields: 16 serving
Total prep & cooking time: 50 minutes + 1 hr. chilling time
Nutrition Facts: Calories: 188 | Protein: 3.4 g | Net Carbs: 2.4 g | Fat: 17.5 g

What to use:

The Crust:

- Almond flour (1.25 cups)
- Swerve Sweetener (.33 cup)
- Salt (.25 teaspoon)
- Melted butter (.25 cup)

The Filling:

- Unchilled cream cheese (3 ounces - softened)
- Lime zest (2 teaspoons)
- Sugar-free condensed milk (1 cup)
- Egg yolks (4)
- Key lime juice (6 tablespoons)
- Also Suggested: 8 by 8-inch baking pan

What to do:

1. The Crust: Warm the oven to 325° Fahrenheit/163° Celsius.

2. Whisk the almond flour with salt and sweetener.
3. Melt the butter and add to the mixture to make the batter.
4. Pour the batter into the pan. Press firmly into the bottom.
5. Bake until just golden brown around the edges (for 12-15 min.).
6. Transfer to the countertop to cool.
7. The Key Lime: Beat the cream cheese and lime zest until creamy smooth.
8. Whisk and fold in the egg yolks until well mixed.
9. Slowly pour in the juice from the lime and condensed milk. Stir until the filling is creamy smooth.
10. Add the filling into the crust. Bake it for 15-20 minutes.
11. Remove and cool. Store in the fridge for at least one hour to set.
12. Top with lightly sweetened whipped cream and lime slices if desired.

Lemon Fat Bombs

Like our other fat bombs, these are no-bake, simple, fantastic, and use only a handful of ingredients.

Yields: 16 servings
Total prep & cooking time: 40 minutes
Nutrition Facts: Calories: 114 | Protein:0.9 g | Fat: 11.9 g | Net Carbohydrates: 0.8 g

What to use:

- Coconut butter (0.75 cup - melted)
- Coconut oil (.5 cup, melted)
- Fresh lemon juice (3 tablespoons)
- Your preferred liquid sweetener (15 drops)
- Lemon zest (1 tablespoon)

What to do:

1. Mix each of the ingredients in a mixing container until they are well-combined.
2. Place the mixture into molds, an ice cube tray, or another container. Put this in the fridge for about ½ hour or until it's set. These keep best in the fridge.

Magical Chocolate Chip Bars

Yields: 16 servings
Total prep & cooking time: 45 minutes
Nutrition Facts: Calories: 132 | Protein: 1.8 g | Fat: 12.4 g | Net Carbohydrates: 6.9 g

What to use:

- Preferred sweetener (or stevia) (2 tablespoons)
- Almond flour (1.5 cups)
- Coconut oil (melted) (3 tablespoons)
- Salt (0.25 teaspoon)
- Walnuts (finely chopped) (0.25 cup)
- Mini chocolate chips (.75 cup)
- Canned coconut milk (1.25 cup)
- Shredded coconut (.66 cup)
- Cocoa powder (optional but encouraged) (2 tablespoons)

What to do:

1. Ensure your oven is allowed time to preheat to 350° Fahrenheit/177° Celsius.
2. Cover an eight-inch pan thoroughly using parchment paper - ensuring the parchment paper goes up the sides of the pan slightly. Set to the side for later use.
3. Toss the almond flour, sweetener, salt, and oil in a mixing container to form a thick mixture. Press this mixture into the parchment-lined baking pan, being careful to press it down evenly.
4. Sprinkle the coconut, nuts, and chocolate chips over the top of the pressed mixture.
5. Combine the cocoa powder and coconut milk in a bowl, whisking thoroughly, and then pour the mixture into the pan to cover the other ingredients.
6. Place the pan into your preheated oven and allow it to bake for ½ hour.
7. Transfer it to a cooling rack for 15 minutes before slicing.
8. Once cool, slice the bars and remove them from the pan. If you would prefer firmer bars, refrigerate them overnight to give them a chance to firm up.

Mint Chocolate Chip Vegan Ice Cream

This ice cream is a great and easy stand-in for dairy ice cream and is vegan and keto-friendly. You also don't need to churn or knead or use an ice cream maker - it's super easy!

Yields: 2 servings
Total prep & cooking time: 2 hours and 15 minutes (largely unattended)
Nutrition Facts: Calories: 151 | Protein: 1.5 g | Fat: 15 g | Net Carbohydrates: 3.5 g

What to use:

- Full-fat coconut milk (1 cup)
- Avocado (about 0.3 of a whole avocado)
- Lemon juice (.5 teaspoon)
- Peppermint extract (0.5 to 0.75 teaspoon)
- Vanilla extract (.5 teaspoon)
- Powdered sweetener of your choice (2 to 4 tablespoons, or more if you want it sweeter)
- Mini chocolate chips or cacao nibs (0.25 to 0.3 cup)

What to do:
1. Put the coconut milk, vanilla extract, peppermint extract, avocado, lemon juice, sweetener, and salt into a food processor - blend these ingredients till they become creamy.
2. Put ice cream in a sealable container and place it in the freezer until the ice cream is set. (This should take about two hours, depending on the size of the container you have chosen.) If you freeze it overnight, it needs to sit at room temperature for between 10 and 20 minutes before serving; otherwise, it will be too hard to easily
eat.

Peanut Butter Truffles

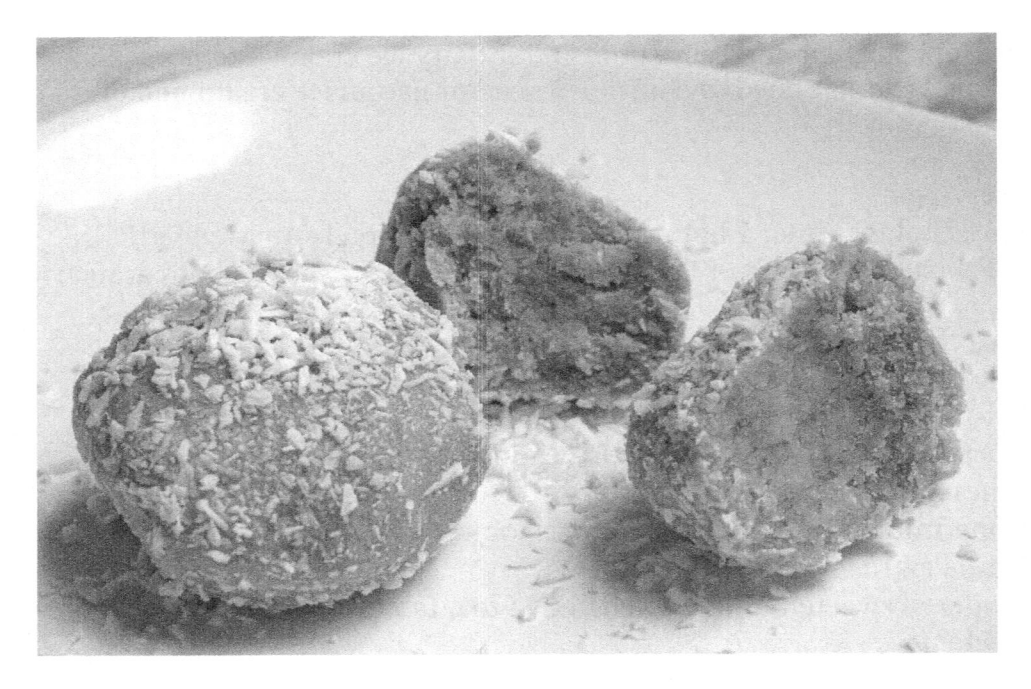

These truffles are so easy to make - just a few ingredients and no baking required!

Yields: 12 truffles
Total preparation & cook time: 1½ hours (largely unattended)
Nutrition Facts: Calories: 110 | Protein: 4 g | Fat: 9 g | Net Carbohydrates: 4 g

What to use:

- Creamy peanut butter (.5 cup, unsweetened, plain peanut butter works best)
- Powdered sweetener of your choice (0.33 cup, to mimic confectioner's sugar)
- Blanched almond flour (0.25 cup)
- Baking chocolate (3 ounces, unsweetened)
- Powdered sweetener of your choice (3 tablespoons, to mimic confectioner's sugar)
- Coconut oil (1 tablespoon)

What to do:

1. Combine the peanut butter, ⅓ cup of powdered sweetener, and ¼ cup of blanched almond flour to a bowl and mix well until these ingredients form a sort of dough.
2. Cover a baking tray thoroughly and completely with parchment baking paper. Form peanut butter mixture into 12 1" balls.
3. Put the tray into the freezer for a minimum of half an hour. Being frozen will make it easier to dip in the chocolate.

4. Combine the chocolate, three tablespoons of powdered sweetener, and coconut oil in a bowl. Microwave the mixture using 30-second intervals, mixing well in between. Don't overheat the chocolate, or it will scorch.
5. Remove the peanut butter balls from the freezer. Use toothpicks to lift them and dip them in the chocolate mixture. Coat the peanut butter ball in chocolate and put it back on the baking sheet.
6. Once all peanut butter balls have been coated, put the baking sheet in the fridge until the chocolate hardens (about an hour). These keep best in the fridge.

Protein Shake - Chocolate

This shake doesn't require any protein powder - all the protein is naturally found in the shake's ingredients. It's also an incredibly simple breakfast or mid-afternoon drink.

Yields: 1 serving
Total prep & cooking time: 5 minutes
Nutrition Facts: Calories: 440 | Protein: 15.6 g | Fat: 31.2 g | Net Carbohydrates: 8.2 g

What to use:

- Almond milk (.75 cup)
- Ice (.5 cup)
- Cocoa powder - unsweetened (2 tablespoons)
- Your preferred sugar substitute (2 tablespoons, but if you like it sweeter, add more!)
- Almond butter (2 tablespoons)
- Hemp seeds (2 tablespoons)
- Chia seeds (1 tablespoon)
- Salt (a pinch)
- Vanilla extract (.5 tablespoon)

What to do:

1. Toss each of the fixings into a food processor - blend until they are a smooth consistency.
2. Pour the resulting smoothie into a glass, serve, and enjoy!

Vegan Chocolate Fudge

This fudge will melt in your mouth! It's super easy and only takes a few minutes to prepare.

Yields: 12 pieces
Total prep & cooking time: 5 minutes
Nutrition Facts: Calories: 97 | Protein: 0 g | Net Carbs: 2 g | Fat: 10 g

What to use:

- Cocoa powder (0.5 cup)
- Full-fat coconut milk (0.25 cup)
- Coconut oil (0.5 cup, melted)
- Vanilla extract (0.5 teaspoon)
- Almond extract (1 teaspoon)
- Your preferred liquid sweetener (2 teaspoons or 20 drops of liquid stevia)
- Salt (a pinch)

What to do:

1. Thoroughly mix all of the ingredients.
2. Drop the resulting mixture into ice cube trays, a lined storage container, or a muffin pan with liners. Put in the fridge.
3. Remove from the fridge once the fudge is cool. Remove the fudge from the muffin pan or ice cube tray. If you used a storage container, slice the fudge into serving-sized pieces.
   Store in the fridge and enjoy when you want fudge!

Chapter 10: Keto Basic 21-Day Meal Plan

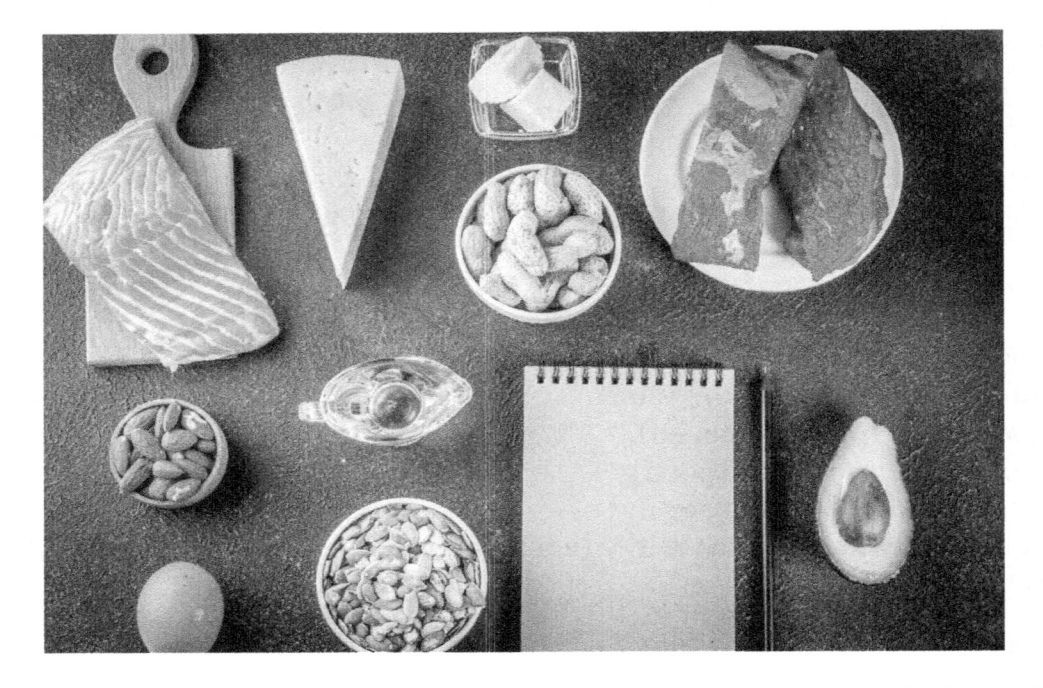

Each day of the meal plan is calculated using the basic 20-25 net carbs daily. Each meal has its counts listed. If you see a meal that is not one desired for that day, simply switch it with one that requires the same amount of nutrients.

Keep in mind, if you want less carbs for a particular day, cut the recipe in half and you are set!

Thanks again for choosing this book, I'd be really happy if you could leave a short review on Amazon, it means a lot for me!

Week One:

Breakfast	Snack	Lunch	Snack	Dinner
Day 1 Healthy Green Smoothie 4 g	Almond snack 1 oz. portion 2 g	Superfood Soup 7g	Chocolate Fat Bombs 5g	Bruschetta Chicken 4g
Day 2 Apple Pie Pancakes 3.5 g	Olives 1 cup 4 g	Arugula Salad with Cherry Tomatoes 1 g	Leftover Chocolate Fat Bombs 5g	Greek Meatballs with Tomato Sauce 12 g
Day 3 Crust-Free Mini Quiche 9.6 g	8 medium strawberries + sugar-free heavy whipped cream 6g	Grab & Go Jar Salad 4 g	Crunchy Protein Bars 5g	Creamy Instant Pot Chicken 9 g
Day 4 Leftover Crust-Free Mini Quiche 9.6 g	Sunflower Seeds ¼ cup portion 2 g	Kale Salad 3 g	Leftover Chocolate Fat Bombs 5 g	Pork Carnitas 1 g
Day 5 Tofu Scramble 8g	Cacao Nibs ⅛ cup or 2 g	Healthy Edamame Kelp Noodles 5 g	Energy Balls 3 g	Mutton Curry 6.34 g
Day 6 Avocado Protein Smoothie 11 g	Pickles Dill-spicy-unsweetened @ Six spears 2 g	Avocado Mint Chilled Soup 4 g	Leftover Energy Balls 3 g	Chipotle Pork Roast 4 g
Day 7 Crumbly Blueberry Bars 6 g	Roll-Up Deli Meat 2 oz. Roasted Turkey + 2 club crackers or cheese -0- g	Grab & Go Jar Salad 4 g	Mint Chocolate Chip Vegan Ice Cream 3.5 g	Pork Ribs 2 g

Week Two:

Breakfast	Snack	Lunch	Snack	Dinner
Day 1 Healthy Green Smoothie 4 g	Cauliflower & Blue Cheese Dip 1 cup caul. + 2 tbsp. dip 3.5 g	Baked Zucchini Noodles With Feta 5 g	Chocolate Avocado Pudding 12 g	Lemon Rotisserie Chicken 2.9 g
Day 2 Cinnamon Roll Muffins 3 g	Radish Chips & Guacamole ½ cup radishes + 2 tbsp. guacamole 5 g	Greek Chopped Salad 2 g	Lemon Fat Bombs 0.8 g	Spicy Pork – Korean Style 9g
Day 3 Cinnamon Roll Muffins 3 g	Tasty Turmeric Milkshake 7 g	Carrot Onion & Beef Soup 3 g	Magical Chocolate Chip Bars 7 g	Shepherd's Pie 4.1 g
Day 4 Low-Carb Maple "Oatmeal" 12.37 g	Avocado - half of 1 + lime squeeze + salt 1 g	Crispy Cauliflower Zucchini Fritters 2 g	Mint Chocolate Chip Vegan Ice Cream 3.5 g	Whole Chicken & Gravy 0.7 g
Day 5 Crumbly Blueberry Bars 6 g	Roll-Up Deli Meat 2 oz. Roasted Turkey + 2 club crackers or cheese -0- g	Delicious Marinara Zoodles 5 g	Protein Shake - Chocolate 8 g	Pork Ribs 2 g
Day 6 Leftover Crumbly Blueberry Bars 6 g	1% Cottage Cheese ½ cup 3 g	Pad Thai with Zucchini Noodles 4 g	Peanut Butter Truffles 4 g	Italian Meatballs 5 g
Day 7 Avocado Protein Smoothie 11 g	Baked Seaweed 1 20-count package 3 g	Chicken "Zoodle" Soup 4 g	Chocolate Avocado Ice Cream 12 g	French Garlic Chicken 4 g

Week Three:

Breakfast	Snack	Lunch	Snack	Dinner
Day 1 Avocado Smoothie with Matcha 4.4 g	Greek Yogurt 6 oz. plain non-fat 7g	Greek Chopped Salad 2 g	Chocolate Fudge 2 g	Steak & Cheese Pot Roast 3.5 g
Day 2 Low-Carb Maple "Oatmeal" 12.37 g	Baked Zucchini Chips 1 g	Carrot Onion & Beef Soup 3 g	Energy Balls 3 g	Pork Carnitas 1 g
Day 3 Crust-Free Mini Quiche 9.6 g	Hard-boiled eggs 1 @ -0- g	Grab & Go Jar Salad 4 g	Key Lime Bars 2 g	Thai-Inspired Peanut Red Curry Vegan Bowl 10 g
Day 4 Overnight Vanilla "Oatmeal" 9.1 g	String Cheese (1) -0- g	Avocado Mint Chilled Soup 4 g	Leftover Key Lime Bars 2g	Creamy Instant Pot Chicken 9 g
Day 5 Tasty Tofu Scramble 8g	Pecans 1 oz. 1 g	Fettuccine Chicken Alfredo 1g	Crunchy Protein Bars 5 g	Beef Stroganoff 6 g
Day 6 Apple Pie Pancakes 3.5 g	Carrot Sticks - 1 cup 8 grams	Kale Salad 3 g	Chocolate Fat Bombs 5 g	Bruschetta Chicken 4 g
Day 7 Healthy Green Smoothie 4 g	Blackberries 1 cup 6 g	Bacon Burger Cabbage Stir Fry 4.5 g	Leftover Chocolate Fat Bombs 5 g	Pad Thai with Zucchini Noodles 4 g

Conclusion

I hope you have enjoyed each portion of the *Keto Diet After 50*. Let's hope it was informative and provided you with all of the tools you need to achieve your goals - whatever they may be.

These are a few of the ways you will benefit the most from whichever diet plan you have chosen.

In theory, the keto approach focuses on two things as a starting point:

- Skipping one meal daily to help eliminate extra carbs.
- Eating under 25 grams of carbs daily is a general guideline that categorizes the majority of people.

How to Begin – Theory 1

Step 1: Choose a non-stressful week to begin the ketogenic diet plan.

Step 2: Purge the pantry and fridge.

Step 3: Restock the fridge and pantry with ketogenic food items.

Step 4: Consider skipping one meal each day. Maybe sleep a little longer and have brunch.

Step 5: Don't exceed your net carbs, and don't limit the fat and protein you consume – initially.

Step 6: Make a routine. Drink a large glass of water with a supplement of ½ teaspoon of MCT oil or two teaspoons of coconut oil.

Step 7: Keep track of your ketone levels.

Two Simpler Approaches to the Start of the Keto Diet Plan

Theory 1: Fast for two days and consume less than 20 g net carbs daily
If you have tried other low-carb diets or intermittent fasting, this is a great way to get into a nutritional ketosis status.

Theory 2: Eliminate desserts, pasta, and bread from your diet. Add healthier carbohydrates such as sweet potatoes. Consume less than 80 grams of net carbs daily for a few weeks. Then, lower the grams a little at a time.

Step 1: Lower Your Carb Consumption

The most crucial element in achieving ketosis is a very low-carbohydrate diet. Your cells typically use sugar/glucose as the primary fuel source, but most of your cells can also use other sources as fuel, such as fatty acids, including ketones.

Once the carb intake is lowered, the insulin hormone levels will decline, which allows the fatty acids to be released from fat storage in your body.

Noted, some individuals need to limit their intake of net carbs to 20 grams daily (net carbs equal total carbs minus fiber), whereas others can remain in ketosis while eating twice that amount. If you can restrict your intake to 20 or fewer grams each day for the first two weeks, you should be guaranteed that ketosis is reached. At that time, you can relax and maintain the ketosis state.

Step 2: Increase the Healthy Fat Intake to Your Diet Plan

Forget the old sayings of it has too much fat. You can help boost your ketone levels by consuming plenty of *healthy* fats. The lowered carbohydrate intake teams up with the high fats to produce ketosis. If you are using the ketogenic diet for weight loss, you can also achieve 60-80% of your calories from your diet's fat. Note, the traditional diet plan for epilepsy is higher, with 85-90% of the calories from fat.

It is important to use high-quality food sources since such a large percentage of your diet is derived from fat intake. Consider using these good fats for your cooking needs; butter, coconut oil, avocado oil, tallow, and lard. You will soon discover how many high-fat foods are low in carbs, but you still need to count them to prevent losing the ketosis state. In general, you should consume a minimum of 60 percent of your daily calories from fat to boost the ketone levels. Make your selections from both animal and plant sources.

Step 3: Include Coconut Oil Into Your Ketogenic Diet Plan

The oil is also used as one of the best methods to improve ketone levels for individuals who suffer from nervous system disorders, such as Alzheimer's disease.

Coconut oil contains medium-chain triglycerides (MCTs), which speed up the ketosis process. Unlike many other fats, the MCTs are absorbed quickly and go directly to the liver, where they are used for immediate energy – resulting in conversion to ketones. The oil contains four types of these fats, 50% of which comes from lauric acid. Continued research has indicated a higher percentage may produce sustained ketosis levels because it is metabolized more gradually than other MCTs. Add coconut oil slowly to your diet because it can cause diarrhea and stomach cramping until you adjust. Begin with one teaspoon daily, and work it up to two to three tablespoons for a week.

Step 4: Maintain Protein Intake

You must supply your liver with amino acids, which can make new glucose (gluconeogenesis). Your liver produces the glucose for the cells and organs in your body that cannot use ketones as fuel - including portions of the brain, kidneys, and red blood cells.

Protein also maintains muscle mass when the carb intake is lowered, especially during a weight loss program. Research has indicated the preservation of your muscle mass and physical performance is at maximum speed when the intake range is 0.55-0.77 grams per pound of lean mass.

Think of it simply; excessive protein intake may suppress ketone production, whereas consuming too little can lead to muscle mass loss.

Step 5: Test the Ketone Levels & Adjust the Diet Plan

Maintaining ketosis is an individual process, and you need to be sure you are achieving your goals. The acetone, acetoacetate, and beta-hydroxybutyrate levels can be measured by your breath, blood, and urine.

You can use a '*Ketonix*' meter to measure your breath. You breathe into the meter. The results will be provided by a special coded color that will flash to show your ketosis levels at that time.

Measure the ketones with a blood ketone meter, which works similarly to a glucose meter. Add a small drop of blood on a testing strip and insert the tab into the meter. It will indicate the amount of beta-hydroxybutyrate in your bloodstream. This process has been researched as a valid indicator of the current ketosis levels. Unfortunately, the strips are expensive.

Test your urine for acetoacetate. The strip is dipped into the urine, which will change the color of the strip. The various shades of purple and pink indicate the levels of the ketones. The darker the color on the testing strip, the higher the level of ketones. The significant benefit is they are inexpensive. The most effective time to test is early in the morning - after a ketogenic diet dinner the evening before testing.

You should use one or more of these methods to indicate whether you need to adjust your intake of foods to remain in ketosis.

Lastly: Bring A New Set Of Rules At The Table

Skip the highest ranks of GPS – grains, potatoes, and sugar.

Focus on veggies, fats, and proteins. Visit a restaurant that offers a healthy salad bar, seafood spreads, carving stations, and vegetable platters. You can usually find butter, olive oil, sour cream, and cheese in plentiful supply.

Use a smaller plate. Play a mind game and fill a small plate instead of a larger one. Try it; this works.

Take your time. Enjoy your time spent with the conversation of a friend or family member. Drink your water and sip your tea or coffee. Enjoy and feel satisfied!

Make Wise Drink Decisions: The best choice is water, tea, coffee, or sparkling water. Decaf coffee or herbal tea is another excellent option. If alcohol is your craving, choose dry wine, champagne, or light beer. Also, consider spirits – straight or with a bit of club soda.

Choose Dessert Wisely: If you are still hungry, try to have another cup of tea or a cheese platter. Have a portion of berries with heavy cream. What about some cream in your coffee?

These are a few more recommendations that might help:

- *Breakfast Suggestions:* Sometimes, there is nothing better than eggs if you want to play it safe. You may be off on some of the counts, but after some practice, you will know how to gauge your eating habits for the most important meal of the day.

- *Lunchtime Suggestions:* Chicken and fish are usually good choices. Many of the restaurants now offer diet-friendly menus. Select a chicken salad or a regular salad. Just be cautious of the dressing used. Try some vinaigrette or plain vinegar.

- *Dinner Suggestions:* Always choose a fresh green veggie with a lean cut of meat as your main course. Try something in the hamburger line minus the bun or a tempting entrée of broccoli and steak.

These are just for starters!

Finally, if you found this book useful in any way, a review on Amazon is always appreciated! Thank you.

Made in the USA
Coppell, TX
16 September 2021